A Year in My Shoes

A Year in My Shoes

✦

A Cancer Survivor's Story

Louise Lampard

Foreword by Dr Corinne Doll BSc MD FRCP(C)

iUniverse, Inc.
New York Lincoln Shanghai

A Year in My Shoes
A Cancer Survivor's Story

iUniverse books may be ordered through booksellers or by contacting:

iUniverse
2021 Pine Lake Road, Suite 100
Lincoln, NE 68512
www.iuniverse.com
1-800-Authors (1-800-288-4677)

Because of the dynamic nature of the Internet, any Web addresses or links contained in this book may have changed since publication and may no longer be valid.

The views expressed in this work are solely those of the author and do not necessarily reflect the views of the publisher, and the publisher hereby disclaims any responsibility for them.

ISBN: 978-0-595-46081-6 (pbk)
ISBN: 978-0-595-70586-3 (cloth)
ISBN: 978-0-595-90380-1 (ebk)

Printed in the United States of America

For my wonderful husband Martin. Without his constant love and support I don't know how I would have survived the most traumatic year of my life. Martin, thank you and I love you with all my heart.

Man can live for forty days without food,
three days without water,
eight minutes without air but only one second without hope.
Bill Cosby.

Contents

Foreword by
Dr. Corinne Doll BSc, MD
FRCP(C)

I first met Louise and her husband Martin in the outpatient department of the cancer centre to discuss radical radiotherapy treatment. As a young woman recently diagnosed with cancer, she was obviously fearful and uncertain of what the future would hold.

However, by the end of that visit, her demeanor had changed. It became obvious to me that here was a very strong woman, with a very supportive husband, who was prepared to do whatever it took to get well.

Louise decided it was important for her, to get through the daily treatment uncertainties and hurdles, to document her experiences and daily discoveries through diaries and emails. This book is the result of Louise's efforts to put pen to paper, or fingers to keyboard—initially for her own emotional healing, but ostensibly to assist others in their own journeys from diagnosis through treatment to recovery and healing. Each patient's experience with cancer therapy is unique; however Louise's frankness, humor and willingness to reveal vulnerability at a time when "a stiff upper lip" may be more accepted by others, illustrates what real patients on treatment go through. The journey is one of strength and hope. The load is lightened by the support of loving family and friends.

This "Platinum Girl" has not only become an advocate for cancer patients, but an active participant and motivator in fund-raising activities for cancer research and treatment. Her ability to take a negative situation, face it bravely, and turn it into something positive for herself and others is something we can all learn from.

Acknowledgments

First and foremost, I would like to say thank-you to Dr Corinne Doll for saving my life.

A huge thank you also to my husband, Martin for his unwavering support and total belief in my recovery—you made the journey so much more bearable.

I will be forever grateful to the staff at the Tom Baker Cancer Centre for their compassion and friendship, John, Salima, Kleve & Doreen from the radiation unit, Glenda, Carleen and Robbi from the chemotherapy ward and Donna, Sheru and Judy, Dr Doll's amazing nurses.

The following people helped me in my hour of need; I am both proud and grateful to be able to call you friends, James & Joanne Green Mead, Clint & Andrea Undseth, Karen Freeborn, John & Melissa Neumann and Maureen Kew.

I would like to say a special thank-you to someone who probably doesn't realize that she had such a profound effect on my life and on my recovery, the lady who talked to the fish, Constance O'Laughlin.

Lastly but by no means least, I would like to thank my mum Margaret.

Introduction

My story really starts in April 2002 when my husband was diagnosed with testicular cancer.

We were living in southern England, enjoying a 'dinky' lifestyle—double income, no kids—when Martin contracted a urinary tract infection. After several courses of antibiotics and numerous visits to the doctor's office, we were finally referred to a specialist.

Our meeting with the urinary surgeon went well initially, he outlined all of the tests that Martin would be having, none of them sounded pleasant but we were relieved that hopefully something was going to be done to put an end to Martin's discomfort.

After the initial examination, Dr H advised that Martin did indeed have a prostate infection that was notoriously difficult to get rid of. He suggested that we were not to worry, he could be cured but it would just take a while. He sent Martin to have the remainder of his tests done at the ultrasound department and said he would talk to us about medication after he had seen the scan results.

When Martin joined me outside the doctor's office after his scan, he was white as a sheet. He described the tests that he had just endured and then said that he knew something serious was wrong. I didn't believe him at first but he insisted that the ultrasound technician had mentioned a tumour.

Dr H called us back into his office and as we sat down he said "Mr Lampard, you are a very lucky young man, we have found a tumour on your right testicle, if you hadn't seen us about your infection, we would never have found this so early."

I remember crying a lot, I was devastated that my partner and best friend, had cancer. Martin was much more practical, when we got home has asked me to call his mum, my mum and his sister, he didn't want anyone else to know. He spoke to the human resources department where he worked and arranged to get the time off that he needed. Within a week, he was admitted to hospital to have the tumour removed and was booked to have a dose of Carboplatin chemotherapy the following month.

We decided to get married in order to ensure that we were each others next of kin. At that time we have been together for almost a decade but had previously never felt the need to get married. Two weeks after Martin's chemotherapy, on July 26th 2002, we tied the knot during a civil ceremony with just two friends, Esther and Kim, present as our witnesses.

Soon after our wedding, we started discussing how we could improve our life and eliminate the stress that we saw as having caused Martin's cancer. We decided that our careers would have to end as they were the main contributor of major stress in our lives. Our only option, if we were to no longer work, would be to emigrate. I had lived in Canada some years before and we both loved the people and the lifestyle available to us. Also the country was vast, we loved skiing and the outdoors so as soon as Martin was well enough, we put our house up for sale and prepared to move half way around the world.

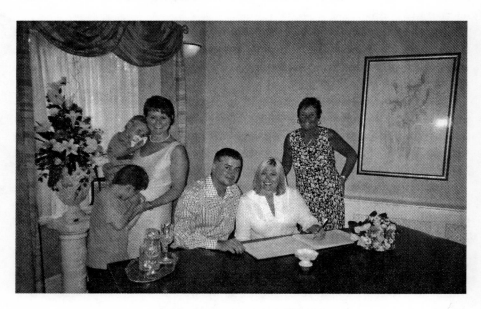

Our wedding day, July 26th 2002

1

The Diagnosis

The day of my cancer diagnosis was almost a relief; the build up to that day had been horrendous.

Four months earlier I noticed a small amount of blood in my underwear, my period wasn't due for over a week and I was usually very regular. I really don't recall giving the incident much thought, after all I always had my pap smear done on a regular basis, the following month however, the same thing happened and I mentioned it to my husband. We had had a pretty stressful few months; we had given up successful careers and our home in the UK to move to Canada, so we kind of blamed stress but decided to visit the doctor once our latest batch of visitors left.

As we were still fairly new immigrants we hadn't found a family doctor so had to use the local walk in clinic. I explained the situation and my symptoms to the doctor and also informed him that twenty years earlier my mother had been diagnosed with cervical cancer although at this point I truly thought I had some sort of infection that would disappear with a course of antibiotics!

The doctor insisted that there was probably nothing wrong with me and eventually after a lot of persuading, agreed to make me an appointment for the following week so he could do a Pap smear. As luck would have it my period started and it was a further two weeks before I could get back to the surgery. Dr L was obviously a busy man and tried to usher me out of his office without doing the smear—he was insistent that my problems were all in my mind and it was at that point that I cried and my husband stepped in to insist that the doctor perform the Pap test.

As soon as the doctor inserted the speculum I started to bleed very heavily, the doctor said that I shouldn't have come to see him when I had my period, I told him that this wasn't a period but he got up and left the room, telling me to clean up so he could come back and talk to me. I was clearly distraught and my husband cleaned up the table and floor whilst I tried to compose myself. When Dr L came back he suggested that it was somehow my fault that he couldn't complete the smear test and although he said he wanted me to visit a gynecologist, it would be impossible to make me an appointment without a current Pap result. We were at a horrible stalemate. I was now very upset and had convinced myself that I probably had cancer. The doctor said he would call us in a couple of days to see how I was and I should go home and not worry!

Back at home, Martin ran a bath for me and just as I got in it the phone rang. It was the nurse at the doctor's office, she explained that she could obviously tell that I was worried and felt that the quickest way to get the matter resolved would be to visit the local emergency room because the sooner I 'got in the system' the sooner I could get an appointment with a gynecologist. She said she would fax a letter to the local emergency room and we needed to get there as soon as possible.

The emergency room wasn't very busy and I was lucky to be seen fairly quickly. I was still bleeding quite heavily and a nurse was assigned to look after me. A doctor came to see me and did an internal exam. She said that she wanted to get a second opinion but thought that I had fibroids—a non malignant, harmless tumor—a second doctor entered the room and managed to take a swab for a Pap smear, he also carried out a pelvic examination. I was by now experiencing quite a bit of abdominal pain and was still bleeding quite heavily, I was desperate to go home but the doctor wouldn't release me until an appointment had been made for further investigations to be done. The gynecologist that I needed to see was about to take a two week holiday and had agreed to see me on her return as long as the hospital provided her with my current Pap results. The hospital finally discharged me at 1am very tired and sore but relieved that 'all I had' were fibroids.

Over the next few days I researched fibroids extensively on the internet, although my symptoms were similar to that diagnosis, they were also similar to another diagnosis that kept cropping up—cervical cancer.

A friend of mine, Kim, arrived for a visit from the UK, her sons, Jamie and Daniel, are like my own children so my mind was taken off of my worries for a while as the boys kept us occupied playing in the local lake every day. In the course of discussing my symptoms with Kim, I somehow managed to convince myself that I must surely have fibroids.

Only three years earlier aged 40, my husband had been diagnosed with testicular cancer; he had endured a major operation and one very high dose of chemotherapy, so between us we had decided it would be very unlikely that we would both be unlucky enough to have cancer at such a young age!

We came to the ridiculous conclusion that if I could have a hysterectomy which would remove the fibroids, I would be fine; little did I realize how wrong I was.

Four weeks passed with no word on my appointment with Dr M. I telephoned the emergency room to see if they had any other information. The nurse looked up my file and realized that it had accidentally been put away without anyone making my follow up appointment. She arranged for me to visit the gynecologist at the first available slot in three days time. The gynecologist's office contacted me almost immediately to inform me that I would be having a colposcopy examination and probably a biopsy as well. Up until this point I was still fairly convinced that I had fibroids and was very nervous about having a biopsy as I have such a low pain threshold.

Whilst I was on the phone, I asked the nurse if she had the results of my smear test that had been done at the hospital, she looked at my file and informed me that my Pap smear was indeed abnormal and I had very high dysplasia. I just knew that I had cancer. I had taken the call whilst at work and as I finished my conversation I just started to cry. James, my employer, sent me home and I called Martin to tell him that I was on my way, I could hardly see through my tears but managed to get home safely where I collapsed into Martin's arms. We decided to go out for a drive mostly because we didn't know what else to do. We drove into the mountains but didn't really talk much, one minute I was convinced I would be fine and the next, I was in floods of tears. It was a very difficult day and a long wait over the weekend until my gynecologist appointment.

It was my 35th birthday that weekend and we both hoped that some time away would stop the worrying and maybe help to pass the time more quickly. We stayed in a lovely hotel in Kimberley, British Columbia, but all weekend the only subject that we could think about or talk about was cancer.

Tuesday arrived, and although I was very nervous I really wanted to get the appointment over with. At this point we hadn't told any friends or family about our concerns so we were carrying the weight of the world on our shoulders. Once we arrived at the hospital, I was very reluctant to go inside and found myself dragging along behind Martin, feeling very nervous and wishing I was somewhere else. We checked in at the front desk and the nurse told us that we had to have a chat about the procedure before the biopsy was taken. She took us into a small room and started to explain Pap smear results in general. I got a bit upset and Martin told her that I was scared that I had cancer because of what I had been told about my smear test result. My results were in the nurse's folder and she took them out and said although the test showed very high dysplasia she had no reason to believe that I had cancer at all. I asked her "if I had cancer would that show on my results?" and she said it would definitely show up as cancer. I can't tell you in that moment, how my emotions changed from such a low to an almighty high. I could barely believe what I was hearing—it couldn't possibly be cancer, the nurse had just assured me. We had spent so long being so worried over nothing at all, I wanted to laugh out loud, I felt amazing and so, so relieved. We kept smiling at each other and although I was still nervous about the biopsy, I was also suddenly fearless.

Dr M called us into her office, I was asked to put on a hospital gown and get up onto the bed. Martin held my hand and the doctor introduced herself and asked if I knew what a colposcopy was. I said that I knew that she was going to take a sample of tissue from my cervix and that I was very nervous, mostly because I had such a low pain threshold. My legs were shaking so badly that a nurse had to hold them still. There were some lovely posters of beaches on the ceiling and I remember laughing when the doctor said she was finished, it didn't hurt at all. I sat up and watched Dr M writing her notes, as she looked up at me, my world fell apart.

She said that although my biopsy would still have to be sent to the lab for analysis, she was 99.9% sure that I had cancer. She said that she had never been more certain of a diagnosis without lab confirmation. I remember screaming "I knew it, I knew it was cancer" and then I looked at Martin, I thought he was going to faint. The color had drained from his face and he just sat with his head in his hands. I got dressed and we were ushered into another room. Someone brought us a glass of water and scheduled us an appointment for that Friday to discuss the biopsy results. A nurse asked us if we had any faith or wanted to see a priest! I could have punched her, I wanted to go straight home and kill myself.

Somehow we made it home and I called my sister and then my best friend Jo. It was 1am in England and although I felt bad waking them up, I needed to speak with my friends. Jo was amazing; she said all the right things although I can't now remember exactly what they were! Martin was just devastated and just seeing the look on his face reduced me to tears. He had been so calm when he was diagnosed with his cancer three years previously but now it seemed he couldn't take in the information. An appointment had been made for us to find out the biopsy results in three days time—another grueling wait.

My mum was due to arrive from England for a two week visit and I wanted her to know what was going on before she arrived so she could be strong for us and help us through the next few months. I asked my sister to tell my mum face to face as I knew the diagnosis would devastate her and being epileptic, I was also worried that the stress might bring on a fit. It was also around this time that I decided that we needed some support and I emailed all of our friends in our email contacts list, asking them for their help.

I decided to email my 'support friends' as they became known, at least once a week with an update of treatments, feelings and general news. My first email was very difficult to write and reading the responses was very upsetting.

2

The Return of Big C

Sent: Thursday Aug 25 2005
Subject: The Return of Big C

Hello everyone,

I hope you are all keeping well. We have now been in Canada for almost 1 year (Sept 9th) and for the most part, have had an amazing time.

For those of you who I haven't yet contacted, sorry for telling you this news via email, two days ago I was diagnosed with cancer.

You all know that we have overcome this disease before with Martin and we fully expect to do the same for me. We are obviously still in shock and I really have never been so scared in all my life.

Being so far away from friends and family at a time like this is really hard so I thought I would set myself up with a little internet circle of people that I can rely on to share my thoughts with and who can help to keep us both in a positive frame of mind.

If you would rather not receive my weekly rants and updates, please let me know, I really won't be offended and will remove you from the list.

My treatment will start next week with Dr M. I am going into the Tom Baker Cancer Centre (if any of you knows who Tom Baker is—please let me know!) for investigative surgery to find out where the cancer has spread to—it is currently in my cervix and probably also in my uterus.

Once the doctors know what they are dealing with, I will have a radical hyster-ectomy (for the men on my email list that just means they take away all the downstairs girl bits!!!!)

Chemo and radiotherapy will only be given if the cancer has spread to the pel-vic wall area so fingers crossed everyone.

That's really all the news that we have at the moment. We have decided to stay here in Canada, partly because things are already moving for me on the medical front and partly because we still love it! My mum arrives on Monday and will stay for as long as we need her, so we are not totally on our own.

Please send positive happy emails whenever you feel like it and I will be in touch soon.

Love to everyone

Louise & Martin

Martin found it very hard to accept my decision to let everyone in on our situation; he had reacted to his own cancer very differently and only told people who needed to know. He was however supportive in my choice and agreed that I should do whatever made me feel better.

I was so scared that I couldn't sleep at all and got the shakes when bedtime arrived. Martin moved our bed downstairs to the lounge so that we could fall asleep watching movies. During the day I could tell myself that these days, doctors are so amazing, and they can perform miracles, I'm sure I will be fine. But during the night my sole thought was 'I don't want to die yet'.

My legs would shake violently all by themselves and I would just cry and cry about wanting to live. The odd thing about that is I was also very pre occupied with committing suicide. On a number of occasions, I asked Martin if we should just take some pills and end it all. I never did contemplate taking my life on my own; my thoughts always, rather selfishly, included Martin dying with me.

Looking back it was clear that these thoughts are experienced by most people diagnosed with cancer, the hospital admission forms even asked how often suicidal thoughts have entered your head!

What follows are the responses I received to that first e-mail.

3

Doctor Who?

Kim
Subject: Re: The Return of Big C

Been thinking of you lots & glad to see you are doing positive things. Take it your mum has been brought up to speed from what you say in your email. What day do you go in to hospital?

I told the boys, I think Jamie understands a little about what you're going through but its difficult making a five year old understand. So if you speak to Daniel and he refers to spots on the inside of your tummy like he had on the outside recently when he had chicken pox, you'll know how I tried to explain it to him! They know you have to go in to hospital and it's serious.

Gary is taking Jamie on an outdoor pursuit thingy with the focus football boys next week in Wales for a few days & they go back to school on the 7th.

Louise, you're made of strong stuff & will get through all this, life is not fair I know but don't let the bastards get you down as they say. We're all here if you need us. Don't be afraid to lean on us if you need to.

Lots of love Kim x

I had worked for Kim, looking after her boys, for the nine years previous to our emigration. The boys were like my own sons and I kept worrying that I would have to say goodbye to them before I died. They were great, as children normally are, chatting away about school & friends and generally keeping my mind off of my problems.

Jayne
Subject: Re: The Return of Big C

Hi Louise

Thanks for the e-mail. Sorry to hear your news, I can't believe it after everything you went through with Martin. It's a cruel world.

You bloody e-mail me anytime you like. And if you ever feel low and need a chat, call me. You've got my mobile, but the home number is +44xxxxxx, whatever time of day or night and I mean that from the bottom of my heart.

Your Doctor seems to have things under control, so lots of positive thoughts for you to keep your spirits up will be coming your way.

Tom Baker, by the way, played Doctor Who and is now the narrator on Little Britain. (Doctor Who with brown curly hair and very long colorful scarf that had been knitted for him by his Nan). It's probably someone totally different who has never been in Doctor Who in his life.

I can't believe you've been gone a year. How time flies. Just think of all the wonderful things you've done in that year and all the other things you've yet to do and will do!! You are a strong woman Louise; supporting Martin the way you did proves it. Leaving the UK to start a new life in a foreign country proves it, you're a fighter and you just have to be strong for you now!!! I know I'm a long way away but if there is anything I can do, however small, just let me know.

Anyway, Louise, you take lots of good care of yourself, I'll have you in my thoughts.

Lots of love

Jayne xxxxx

Steve & Kerry
Subject: RE: The Return of Big C

Hi Louise and Martin,

My god terrible news our thoughts and hearts go out to both of you. If there is anything I can do for you then please don't hesitate to ask I have suggested to your mum that I will sort her computer problem out she only has to ask me.

I was hoping to contact you by phone, just got your number from your mum. It would be great to talk to you both soon. We are all well and on holiday in Australia in Sydney as I type.... Don't know if you have SKYPE on your PC great free way of talking all you need is headset with mike and you can make free calls over the internet as long as you are on broadband. You can download it for free from www.skype.com my skype name is ***** look for me and we could talk. Got some great pictures of the weather you sent and have one as a screen saver on my desktop. Glad you're staying in Canada as you worked so hard to get there, and I think it's where your hearts are now. Take care the both of you and hopefully will talk soon on skype or by phone.

Love Steve Kerry Danielle Jessica and of course Joe, oh yes Sam, two rabbits, two gerbils, two chinchillas, whiskers the cat, Mr. Snake and the seven tortoise and twenty 2 fish thinks that's it oh no nearly forgot the two hamsters bye for now xxxxxxxxxxxxxx

James and Michele
Subject: RE: The Return of Big C

Louise:

Thanks for including us.

For everyone else, here is a picture of Louise and our daughter Simone—who is 3. We expect to be taking more pictures of Louise, Luc and Simone in our home, in the near future.

The story behind this picture—Simone made us make a special trip back to the shops at the Jasper Park Lodge, during a trip there last weekend. We had bought her a present at a store and she wanted to get the 'exact same' present for Louise.

Michele, James, Simone & Luc

Unfortunately permission was not given for the bear slipper picture to be included in this book; you'll have to use your imagination!

Kevin & Carol
Subject: Hi

Louise,

Was just in touch with Kim catching up and she gave me your news, just wanted to let you know we are all thinking of you.

Carol's friend in Holland just went through the same recently and all worked out ok.

Kev.

James & Michele were my employers; I worked for them, looking after their two young children. I wasn't able to obtain permission to publish the bear slipper picture from both of them, so I decided to err on the side of caution and leave it out.

Kevin is Kim's brother and over the years I had become good friends with him and his wife, Carol. They immigrated to Australia the same week that Martin & I moved to Canada.

Sue & Keith
Subject; Return of Big C

Well what can we say? I'll keep it short and sweet. How did you find out have you not been well? We wish you lots of luck and love to hope that you both beat this like before, we'd love to hear your updates but I won't constantly keep asking you when we speak or e-mail but you know you can talk whenever you need to.

We went camping on our own this week it was really good. I got the fishing bug and caught three fish. We stayed in a park opposite Santa's Village a theme park where Santa spends his summer the kids thought it was amazing little things and all Mrs. Clause could talk to us about was the Tornado's that came through Fergus.

Last Friday we had two Tornado's come through Fergus (our main small town 15mins away) The devastation was amazing we have never seen anything like it there was no mess then a house with no roof no more mess for a while then on the opposite side of the road tree's were down followed by a barn no mess then a house with a tree resting in the roof. The most amazing thing to see was where in the middle of a forest the trees were all uprooted and snapped like twigs but the surrounding ones didn't even look like they had seen a breeze in days.

One more week and the kids go to school including Paige, YEAH, she is still trying to convince me that I should let her go on the Bus on her first day. Her confidence is amazing Keith, Karl and I would all stand back and Paige would be up front.

Good luck with your Mum coming mine hasn't said when they are coming back if ever. Karl decided to save for a Dirt Bike and when he told my Mum you can imagine her words of encouragement, not.

Anyway must go.

Speak soon. Sue X

Sue and Keith were friends of ours from England; they emigrated two months before us with their children Karl and Paige.

Karen & Peter
Subject: The Return of Big C

I don't know what to say Louise, except life sucks and we are with you one hundred percent girl! I don't want to dwell on sadness as I know this is not going to help at all but if there is anything you guys need or want just ask.

I for one want to be in your support group and am honored that you considered me, so enough of this let's get fighting. You are going to beat this and with this crazy bunch in Canada we'll help you do it, so you are not going to get a chance to be down, I speak from experience believe me, the things they've done to me when I've been low.

Keep us posted Louise,

Love to you both

Karen & Peter xx

Karen became a friend after we moved to Canada, a fellow expat, she was an amazing support during my illness. She emailed me every week, without fail, and really was a tower of strength.

Kay & Graeme
Subject: The Return of Big C

Dear Martin and Louise

I have read and re read, read and re read your message, gone to reply then stopped. Slept on it and are about to try again.... Although Louise" happy positive emails" are a hard call!

I am so sorry and wish you a speedy recovery and am so glad to hear that your mum will be with you both.

I just don't know what else to say to you apart from that I will be thinking of you.

I promise to get to work on the happy positive email soon.

Thinking of you with lots of Love Kay xxxx

Trudi
Subject: The Return of Big C

Hi Louise

I was so shocked to hear from Kim your news, I was in the office when she phoned you. My thoughts are with you and also Martin and I have my fingers crossed that next week goes OK and that the result is not as bad as first forecast. I didn't send you an email immediately because it must be a lot for you both to take in and get your head round.

I thought the picture of you and Simone wearing the same slippers really cute. With lots of love to you both and everything crossed.

Love

Trudi xx

Bill & Pauline
Subject: The Return of Big C

Hi Louise and Martin

Bill and I are so sorry to hear your bad news. But thank goodness the treatments have improved so much now.

I know you must have a multitude of emotions going on right now, but try to stay strong. Our thoughts and love are with you.

Bill tried to phone you last week but you were not in, so he will try again this week. I know he wants to send you an e mail when he gets home from work later, but I wanted to let you know straight away that no matter how far away, we are right there with you in heart.

Keep strong both

All our love

Pauline & Bill

Sue & Jan
Subject: The Return of Big C

Hi Louise,

I am so sorry to hear your very sad news. I am sure that must have knocked you for six, as it would anyone. But you must remain positive, which I am sure is easy for me to say but you will beat it as Martin did. I would continue to be glad to hear how things are going with you.

On a lighter note, I spoke to Jamie last week; he said that he had been out to see you. He was very chatty telling me where he had been and what he had done on his visit to see you. You must have really crammed it all in as they only stayed for a week didn't they? I bet it was great to see them. Did you think that they had grown? Mind you did you say that you speak to them via web cam or whatever it is called? You can see that I'm still not exactly an expert at all this internet lark!

Has Jo been out to see you yet? If so, how did that go?

The children are in Wales at the moment with their dad. Jan and I are going camping for the weekend. At least the weather is scheduled to be ok as it has been horrible recently, more like winter. We decided that unless we actually go away we get so bogged down with doing the limitless jobs that we still have to do on the house. I am sitting at my desk at work today wishing the day away so we can get going.

Anyway, I best go now. Keep in touch. I will be thinking of you.

Take care,

Sue & Jan

Louise & Tony
Subject: The Return of Big C

Hi Louise (and Martin),

So sorry to hear your news.... just can't believe it's happened to you both again.

If ever you need a chat whether it's night or day please call and yes of course include me in your " internet circle of friends" you can rant and rave as much as you like.

I've been doing a Google search for Tom Baker and I found the Cancer Centre, but can't seem to find out who he is (apart from Dr Who). It's bugging me now, I want to know (I'm sad like that).

On a serious note though—as you know I'm not one of this countries biggest fans at the moment so honestly believe that you will get better treatment/service out there than you would get here and having your mum with you as well can only help. Can I ask one question though—how does the health service work out there, I mean is it free like ours or is it similar to the States?

Anyway my thoughts are with you both so take care and I'll speak to you soon. Remember please call anytime or e-mail as I check my inbox regularly.

Lots of love

Louise and Tony xxxxx

MUM
Subject: Re: The Return of Big C

Hi, just read your e-mail I thought I had cried myself dry but obviously not.

I think it's a good idea to keep in touch this way as the time difference won't be such a problem, and people can express themselves better. Everyone here and at work sends love and good wishes, and all are very positive. Alison my boss, said not to worry about work and to take as much time off as I need, so I can stay as long as you need me. I can be strong and positive having been through the same thing, think how much progress there has been in medicine in the 19 years since I was diagnosed.

Love to you and Martin and see you very soon

Mum xxxxx

My mum was very strong throughout my illness. Twenty years previously, she had also been diagnosed with cervical cancer so I guess she knew exactly what I was going through. I wasn't in touch with my dad, although I have since made contact with him. We had fallen out 10 years earlier when he and my mum divorced and both my sister and I had excluded him from our lives. Cancer made me realize that life really is short and I decided to allow my dad to be a part of my life again once I was cured.

Melanie & Jason (my younger sister)
Subject: Re: The Return of Big C

Hi Louise,

The only 'Tom Baker' that Jason and I could think of was the Tom Baker who played Dr. who in the 70's, so I doubt that's who the Centre is named after!

Lots of love

Melanie xxxx

As you can probably tell from this email, my sister is not a woman of many words! I think she found it incredibly difficult to know what to say. Melanie was diagnosed with MS in 1989 and although she generally keeps very well, I was aware that I couldn't really 'lean' on her too much. She was very upset that I was ill but she chose to quietly cheer me on from the sidelines rather than get involved in e-mails.

Aunty Jacky & Uncle David
Subject: Sending lots of love

I have been thinking long and hard as to what platitudes I could make in this e-mail, but really nothing could make better the awful feelings that you and Martin must be having right now, so I'm not going to even try! You do know however, how much Uncle Dave and I are rooting for you and are sending heaps of love from all of us here, so if lots of love and good wishes can be counted you will be sailing through the Hysterectomy and back to your old self in no time. Of course, if you can find anything positive out of all this at the moment just remember no more periods ever again. What a treat that is—believe me take it from one who knows.

I know that your Mum can't get to you quick enough and we have said that we will try to get all the updated news without making ourselves a pain. Too many people keeping on ringing you etc is very exhausting.

Anyway chin up honey and all our positive thoughts are being sent wrapped in a huge great cuddle.

Lots of love to you and Martin

Aunty Jacky and Uncle David

Paul & Dawn
Subject: The Return of Big C

Dear Louise and Martin,

Tom Baker—wasn't he in Dr. Who?
Or am I being a nerd.
Sounds like its time for Martin to give you a big cuddle from us.
I suppose I should send over lots of veggie type stuff, nuts and all.... but I think
you already get a lot of bad winds.... over your way!
1 year on hey!
where does the time go.... got to make Rosie breakfast ... but will write again
soon ...
we will keep our fingers crossed and keep you in our thoughts ...
positive thinking ...
love

Paul, Dawn and Rosie xx

Gemma & Harold
Subject: Hi

Hi Louise,

We are so, so sorry to hear of your bad news. I hope that you're being looked after well and that you make a speedy recovery. We're all thinking of you. :)

It's been a while since I e-mailed so I thought perhaps some mundane chatter from sunny Hampton Court might take your mind off things for a couple of minutes at least! Life has changed drastically since Luis came along—all for the better though! He's 4 months old now and is so lovely. He's got a real funny little personality and certainly knows what he wants. Unless he's asleep though, he demands all of my time and we do try to get out and about and do different things. Next week once the school holidays are over we'll start going to some of the groups again, baby signing, mum & baby group, baby massage ... bla bla bla! It's quite fun and my days fly by. I have started him on solids now and we're doing two small meals a day—way hey!

I won't be going back to work although I haven't told work yet, they assume I'm on leave until May next year. I'm thinking about becoming a registered child minder but we'll see, it depends on what I have to do and what requirements I have to meet! So for the meantime, when I have a spare hour or so (which isn't that often!), I'm becoming a whizz at Ebaying! Soon, we'll have nothing left to sell!

Looking forward to going on holiday very soon. We're going to Cornwall for a week on 10th September and mum and dad are coming too. We're staying in a static caravan on a farm and they're staying in their caravan on the campsite next door—so enough distance if we want it but close enough for the odd spot of babysitting! Mum and Dad are besotted with Luis although Mum's nappy chang-ing skills are a bit rusty. I came back from the hairdressers and she'd changed him and fed him and just as I walked in he did a poo, so I got down to change him and it was a real mess, poo up the back and everything. Mum had only gone and put the disposable nappy on back to front! And they were nappies that had a pic-ture of an animal on the front to indicate which way round the nappy went!

Anyway, I am being yelled at by my son who hasn't had my attention for all of 10 minutes so I won't bore you any further!!

Hope everything goes ok over the next few weeks and we'll be thinking of you!

Take care
Love

Gemma
xxxx

JOHN (Martin's cousin)
Subject: Thinking of you both

Hi Martin and Louise,

I'm lost for words really. I know a couple of friends from work who've had the same form of cancer—it's more common than you might think—and after treatment, they're clear and still around to nag me about being such a fat bastard, so think positive. I'm sure you don't need me to tell you that, after everything you've already both been through, but being a bit of a thicky I thought I'd say it anyway.

The hospitals sound much better than anything we've got over here, where you have to fight off giant cockroaches for bed space. I'm amazed at how quickly your results came through. It seems to be one of the better places to get treatment, which all points towards the best possible outcome.

Anyway, enough of my mutterings please let me know how things are going and remember that there's a fat bastard in Essex wishing you well.

All my thoughts for the best,

John, Mo, Helen & Liam. Xxx

John & Carol
Subject: RE: week 1

Hiya, M & L, sorry I've not replied sooner, due to work I've not opened my e-mails for a fortnight. This is just a quickie to say that our thoughts are with you Louise, and we hope that you're soon back to full strength,100%, pure Louise as soon as possible, with our love & best wishes,

John & Carol

Receiving the many emails that I did was often a pleasant distraction from my life. It showed me that life goes on regardless, whether it was Gemma's toddler keeping her busy or Carol's job preventing her from checking her inbox. The world doesn't stop just because you have cancer.

Elaine
Subject: RE: week 1

I am so very sorry I haven't been in contact and sorry to hear of your recent problems.

The power of positive thinking is a wonder and with your and Martins attitude I think your rapidly on your way to getting through it.

Life really does chuck out some crap to people who really don't deserve it!

I promise I will contact you the weekend and I can keep you up to date with events in my love life.

Yes unbelievable as it sounds I do currently have one!!! And plenty more gossip!

Look after yourself and stay away from the Gin!

Elaine
X

Elaine and I were good friends when I lived in England; our lives took different paths when we subsequently emigrated and I hadn't been it touch very often. As soon as she learned that I was ill however, she contacted me straight away which was nice.

Anita
Subject: Hi

Hi Louise,

I was so shocked to hear your news. Kim told me last week and I am sorry that I haven't been in contact sooner but I have been searching for your e-mail.

It must be difficult for you being out there at a time like this but I am sure that you have the strength and determination to get through this.

Our thoughts are with you

Anita (& Steven) xxx

Anita is Kim's sister, as I had worked for Kim for so long; I had inevitably become friends with her family. Anita was pregnant while I was ill and it was quite nice to have that balance sometimes—her good pregnancy news in trade for my crappy cancer news!

John, Katie & Simon (my cousin)
Subject: Re: cancer week 2

Hiya Louise,

I have just read your first e-mail and I have to say I was quite shocked to hear that you're not well. It seems that when you just get life sorted out and are enjoying life as it's meant to be enjoyed that something awful has to happen to redress the balance. How long is your Mum staying???

You sound pretty positive about things, which is good, I'm sure Martin has a lot to do with that he has got such a good sense of humor and it sounds like he is looking after you very well.

I will be thinking of you over the coming weeks and hope that all goes well with your treatment, it sounds like the hospitals are pretty good out there.

I'm sorry that I didn't reply earlier but we have been away on holiday for most of August, got back and there were a hundred things to do, you know how it is when you get home and then the kids are going back to school. I haven't sat down up here in the study for ages picked up 72 e-mails. Where do they all come from mostly crap?

The Holiday was nice we all flew out to Spain for a couple of weeks and hired a Villa it was a lovely time, Mum came with us as well and enjoyed herself, jumping in the pool, at midnight, at her age, whatever next!!! Thankfully she chose not to go skinny dipping.

Mandy and I went away for a week in a caravan after we got back, just the two of us, no kids it was great.

Back at work now, still hate the job but need the money. Say hello to Martin and Margaret for me.

You take care of yourself and get better soon.

Love

John

Lisa & Rob
Subject: Hi

Hi Louise, sorry it's taken me a while to reply to your email. We have been away on holiday, came back for a few days then went up to Norfolk to sort out the wedding plans. Truth is, when I read your e-mail I couldn't take it all in, I kept thinking back to when we were little and all the things we used to get up to and just couldn't believe it. But it sounds as though you're being really positive and that's good, you can beat this, don't let it get the better of you. I'm sure I told you about my dad, he was diagnosed with cancer two years ago, and he beat it with a positive attitude, healthy diet and a whole heap of determination!!

It's great that your mum is there to support you and obviously you have Martin too. And as for your mum's muffins, well I have the same problem; whenever there is a crisis in the family she bakes trays of them. Actually they are not that bad so I've forwarded the recipe for you!!

Well, thanks for keeping me posted and I really do wish you all the best, let me know all your news as it happens and I'll be as helpful as I can be.

Love Lisa xx

Irene Ianson's muffin recipe
10oz self raising flour—sifted,
a pinch of salt,
3oz dark soft sugar,
3oz margarine,
2oz or more of choc chips and 1 mashed banana
Stir all ingredients together and then beat in 2 eggs with a little milk if necessary but do not make too wet. Bake in middle of oven gas mark 5/190c for about 15/20 minutes or more.

Toni & Derek

Saturday, September 10, 2005

Dearest Louise and Martin,

I have found it extremely difficult to write back, especially as I only got my e-mails yesterday due to holidaying in Italy.

I cannot express the emotional confusion in my mind.

You know the saying don't you "it only happens to the best people", well, now you know why it is a common saying.

On a less miserable note, I am pleased to hear that it hasn't spread and that it can be treated. And as far as having your hair fall out, just imagine never having to say "this job is driving me mad, I'm pulling my hair out!!" ha ha!!

I hope Martin is coping ok, and who else to have around you but your mum, I'm sure she is spoiling you.

My prayers and thoughts will be with you for Wednesday, try not to worry too much (ok for me to say) you are in the best hands.

Love to you all, speak soon.

Toni & Derek. Xxxxxxxxxxxxxxx

We had become friends with Toni & Del just before we left England. Their son James and Jamie (who I looked after) were good friends at school. While it was nice to know that all my friends in England were rooting for me, it felt weird that I couldn't just call in for a coffee of a chat when I wanted to.

From: Sally M
Subject: A short message

Hi Louise,

Its Sally M here, Jo's sister-in-law, hope you don't mind but Jo gave me your e-mail address and I thought I would send you a short message.

I was so sorry to learn that you have cancer, and since James and Jo came back from visiting you in June, Jo has kept me fully informed of your progress. I am pleased that you are beginning treatment in the near future; you must have had a terrible few months what with tests and waiting for results and everything. Still things look positive with the treatment you will have, although I understand there are a few drawbacks.

I have seen the photo's that Jo took when they came to Canada and they look beautiful. When Jo and James told us they were emigrating, I said "where to, Canada?" and was surprised when she said New Zealand. We will miss them all very much, but I don't blame them for going for it! I think it is too easy to look back and say I wish we had done whatever, and good for them for living their dream.

I have only just had this e-mail address set up; my friend's boffin son came round to fix our computer, as he told me it had spy-ware on it (whatever that means! I made out I knew), and while he was here I asked him to set this up for me. I had been asking my two eldest sons' for months but could they be bothered. I have put your address in my favorite's folder along with Jo's; I have had quite a few messages from her already.

Well, I hope this reaches you ok. Please message back if you feel like it.

Take care.

Love Sally.

Sally is the sister in law of my friend Jo. I found that lots of people were interested in my illness and well being, even people that I didn't really know. I had requests from some friends asking if they could pass my emails on to people they knew who were also going through cancer treatments at the same time as me.

Dr Thomas Davidson Baker

(Excerpts from the Eulogy of Dr. Thomas Davidson Baker as delivered by Michael Kostek on May 8th 1997)

Dr. Thomas Davidson Baker was a good man in every sense of the word—a pioneer educator, a humanitarian,—a devoted husband, father and grandfather and a man who made our city and province a better place in which to live. His untiring devotion to duty and his public spirit are attributes, which made him an outstanding leader and one of the great men of Alberta in the 20th century.

Born in Coutbridge, Scotland in 1910, Tom emigrated to Canada as a twelve year old boy. He graduated Calgary Normal school with a first class teacher's certificate in 1928.

Notwithstanding his accomplishments in the tangible aspects of education, Tom Baker served humanity in many other ways—with a special concern for those who had problems. Indeed his name has become synonymous with education for the underprivileged and handicapped.

As a crusader in the fight against cancer, Tom Baker had a tremendous impact on the establishment of diagnostic and treatment services throughout Alberta. For 17 years he served as a chairman of the Provincial Cancer Board and in recognition of this service was named Citizen of the year in 1971 by the Edmonton Chamber of commerce. In 1974, his alma mater the U. of A. conferred upon him the Honorary Doctor of Laws degree.

In 1981, Dr. Baker received yet another high tribute as a new health care facility in Calgary was named the Tom Baker Cancer Centre.

4

Believe That You Will Be Cured

It was very hard to read the wonderful e-mails that my friends had sent. Most people never find out how their friends and family feel about them as usually those sorts of feelings are spoken only at funerals and that is where I felt I was heading. I cried a lot reading them and then made a conscious decision to pull myself together, stop feeling sorry for myself and concentrate on getting better. I planned to e-mail my 'support friends' every week and wrote my e-mails from my heart, never re reading them before I sent them in order to keep them honest.

It becomes very clear when reading the emails that I sent, that I really had no clue what was going to happen to me. I had no idea that the investigations before my treatment could start were so long winded. I obviously appreciate now that of course each individual cancer has to be thoroughly investigated and mapped before treatment can begin, but at the time I think I was assuming that I would turn up for my first hospital appointment and instantly get started on medication.

Getting a cancer diagnosis is the start of a very steep learning curve. There is a very fine line between knowing everything about your cancer and knowing enough to get you through. Among other things, you have to learn to listen to your body, learn to understand medical jargon, have faith in your 'cancer team', stand up for yourself and above all believe that you will be cured.

Subject: week 1
Date: Saturday, August 27, 2005

Hi to all,

Well, give yourselves a big pat on the back and thank you to those of you who had your fingers crossed!

My latest round of tests has shown that the cancer is absolutely NOT in my lymph nodes which basically means that it has not spread far, I am not riddled with it and will not die this weekend at least!

The cancer is however through the whole depth of my cervix and I have abnormal cells in my birth canal (I wasn't aware that I had a birth canal so double shock there!)

Emotionally we are now in a sick kind of way almost pleased that we have some positive news to work with. We explained to Dr M that we didn't want to know or much less dwell on any negative news and certainly don't want to be given survival statistics. I don't want to focus on anything other than being well again.

This week's emotional rollercoaster has been a horrendous ride but I now feel much calmer and don't want to kill myself anymore—I did contemplate doing that on Monday but then realized that Martin (geography genius) probably wouldn't be able to find his way back to the UK without me!

On the bright side, I have lost ten lbs in weight (although I wouldn't recommend cancer as a diet plan!) and Martin is treating me like a queen. He already does most of the cooking and looks after me very well but now I also get massages & foot rubs on request and I haven't had to make so much as a drink in over a week!

We have decided to get back to the healthy diet that we adopted during and after Martin's cancer although this week between us we have consumed a litre of Gin (me), a litre of Brandy (Martin) and between us a large bottle of Bailey's.

Thank you so much for your replies so far, I cried a lot at first but all of them have been so encouraging and it's nice to know that you are all rooting for me.

The next three weeks will be exhausting as I have to go through a lot of different tests although I must say (and this to make the British contingent on my list jealous) I went to get some blood tests done yesterday at the South Calgary medical centre. We showed up at 4.55pm on a Friday, with no appointment and got the tests—results take 2 hours—we were back in the car by 5.05pm!

So clearly the service here in Calgary is much more efficient that at Broomfield or Basildon and even Martin's tests at the Springfield med centre (private hospital—for the Canadians who aren't aware) used to take 10 days!

Well I will sign off now; hope you like the attached picture.

Lots of love Louise xxx

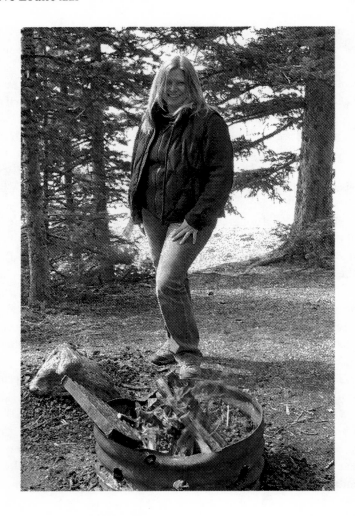

Subject: cancer week 2
Date: Saturday, September 3, 2005

Hi everyone,

well another week goes by & I am starting to get used to the idea that I have this horrible disease! My mum arrived safely and it's been a relief to have her here.

The whirlwind of tests finished yesterday with a CT scan and I am now dreading my Tuesday morning appointment with my oncologist to find out all the results! I had never had a CT scan before but Martin had described to me, what I would feel. The nurse explained the feelings I would get in a very different way.

Nurse's explanation: you will feel warmth in your vagina & will feel like you need to pee.

Martin's explanation: it feels like you've got a hedgehog up your arse!

Although I always feel better after these appointments, I just hate the build up to them. I really think that it would be better if they could just lock you in a room for a day, do all the tests in one go and give you the results immediately!

We have tried to focus this week on the fact that the cancer is not in my lymph nodes but it is hard because every time you get a twinge of pain or even a headache, you can't help thinking that the cancer must have spread and that your life is over!!!

Reading all of your emails has been a great help and every time I feel like crying I read them to cheer myself up. Who knows, maybe I'll write a book one day full of all my messages!

We are going to Millarville farmers market this morning to stock up on fruit & vegetables—mum is looking forward to all the free food samples!!!

Take care & I will send the next e-mail on Tuesday after my appointment when I know what is going to become of me!

Lots of love, Louise xx

Subject: cancer week 2 & half!
Date: Tuesday, September 6, 2005

Well this weekend has flown by, I stubbed my toe on a chair leg and now it has gone black and looks like it's about to drop off—my toe that is, not the chair leg! Like I needed any more problems!

Martin and I went to see Pearl Jam in concert on Sunday night, I think it was just the tonic we needed. The venue (Saddledome in Calgary) was hilarious compared to what we are used to. For the benefit of the Brits who haven't visited us yet—it would be like going to see Robbie Williams at the Cliffs in Southend! We were really close to the stage and seeing Eddie Vedder perform was totally awesome (very Canadian expression!)

I am getting really nervous now about the hospital appt tomorrow. Mum must be as well—she keeps making muffins to keep herself occupied. Typically I have put some weight back on; I was doing so well before on the nervous exhaustion diet plan—ha ha!!!!!

A quick plea to all the Brits—a very good Canadian friend of mine is currently researching the Yorkshire dialect—please send me any useful phrases as she only knows a couple so far![1]

I had a really funny photo sent to me by Tracie and I have attached it because it made me laugh. Also the best piece of advice I got this week was from John—never swallow anything bigger than your head! It has apparently stood him in good stead so I think we should all try to remember that one!

Tuesday morning.

We are getting ready to leave now for the hospital, I am so worried that I am physically shaking—even though I know that the outcome will still be that I have cancer, I am hoping that I hear something positive. Ridiculous as it seems, I am concerned about my hair falling out when I have my treatment! I would never before have described myself as a vain person but I guess I must be—I don't even know for sure that I will have chemo!!!!

We are leaving now so I will write again later.

---

1.   A quick explanation, my Canadian friend Andrea was telling us that her mum was born in Yorkshire, England. We were discussing the various dialects spoken across the country and Andrea offered a hilarious imitation of her mother's accent. I wish that we had recorded the appalling sound that came out of Andrea's mouth—anyone with a Yorkshire dialect would be horrified!

Tuesday afternoon

Just got back from my appointment, my liver, spleen and kidney's are all clear—the cancer if it spreads can touch those organs without going via the lymph nodes so it's a relief to know that all my major organs are ok!

I had a chest x-ray and they took a lot more blood today—just going to weigh myself, surely I must be lighter.… No luck—still weigh the same, oh by the way if anyone has a decent muffin recipe I'd be grateful, mum has been making it up as she goes along and the latest batch were diabolical!

I am going into hospital next Wednesday for the first part of my treatment, it is an investigation under anesthetic and I will be there just for the day. Once the doctor has checked out the area, he will decide if I need chemotherapy or not. The hysterectomy thing is almost certainly on the cards but I am trying not to think about that—I am so squeamish I know I'll pass out if I dwell on it!

Anyway I can at least end this email once again on a positive note.

Lots of love

Louise xx

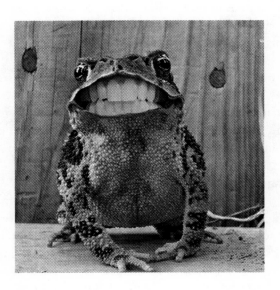

Subject: cancer—week 3 and half!
Date: Tuesday, September 13, 2005
Wednesday morning Sept 7th

Well we sort of celebrated last night as we had got some positive news about my cancer not being present in my lymph nodes, in the morning. We took mum to our local pub; Rip's for fish & chips! Unfortunately as I haven't eaten much lately, I made myself feel really sick by gorging on greasy junk food!

Thursday morning Sept 8th

I feel really panicky today and seem to have lost the ability to make very simple decisions (much to Martin's delight! he thinks he is now in charge!) I am so nervous but not sure what of? We have joined the Sudoku craze that has taken over England and I am trying to keep my head busy with numbers rather than the alternative scary thoughts.

Sunday morning Sept 11th

I woke up today feeling really bad, I can't stop thinking about dying! I think the hardest thing to do is to stay positive when you don't know exactly what you are up against—maybe that will change after Wednesday's appointment although right now, finding out is worse than not knowing I think!

Sunday afternoon

I had a very tearful morning but have managed to rally round this afternoon—mum and Martin are trying to carry on as normal but I know I am making their lives a misery! I feel much better now and am going out for a walk.

Monday morning Sept 12th

I can't believe I feel so great today after such a crappy weekend!!!! I have been so miserable but today I feel fantastic—I got a good nights sleep last night for the first time in ages so that is probably why. Martin has had a cold which is thankfully on its way out and the rain has stopped so we might go out for the day instead of hanging around the house. Martin has taken over from mum & is busy in the kitchen making muffins!!! His are much nicer (much to mum's disgust) I have stopped feeling so angry at everyone maybe that's because I discovered that our local 7-11 store has started selling Cadburys thin chocolate bars!!!!!

Tuesday morning Sept 13th

I am getting nervous now, tomorrow is fast approaching! I am having a good day today, mum has got my sewing machine out so she is in her element & I am trying to find her jobs to do to keep her occupied!! I have had a pedicure & shaved my legs ready for tomorrow—I know it sounds ridiculous but if the doc sees my feet & legs first and they seem looked after, he won't be worried about the other bits he has to look at!!!! Martin has suggested that I may be going mad and I have to say after reading what I have just typed, he may have a point—still roll on tomorrow afternoon and it will all be over—we will know exactly what is going to happen and I can be fixed and get back to normal!

I will e-mail again once I know what is going to happen to me—keep the emails coming, they really cheer me up.

Lots of love Louise xxxx

My being so anxious was compounded by the fact that I had never been in hospital before—I had never ever had stitches, broken a bone or had an anesthetic. As a child I would scream blue murder if I hurt myself in any way and later as an adult I had fainted during blood tests, totally freaked out during a routine visit to the dentist and had to call a nurse on more than one occasion whilst visiting my husband in hospital. To say I was a bit of a baby would be putting it mildly!

Subject: cancer UPDATE!!!!!!!!
Date: Wednesday, September 14, 2005

Hi everyone

Good news today once again—I went into hospital this morning to be 'internally investigated' being put out wasn't nearly as bad as I thought & thanks to all of you who shared your hospital stories, they cheered me up & don't worry, I can keep secrets!!!!!!

I was under anesthetic for about an hour during which time 4 doctors had a good look at my insides to determine exactly where the cancer was.

I had to have a camera put in my bladder—glad I was asleep! And then some poor nurse had to fill my bowel with air—you really don't want to know the consequences of that little number!!!!

So the upshot of all that gross stuff is....

The cancer is not in my bladder or bowel but has spread to a ligament on the left side of the cervix. This means that a hysterectomy cannot be done due to the risk of the cancer spreading if it is cut, so radiation and chemotherapy treatment will be performed daily for the next 7-8 weeks then a 2 day stay in hospital to have internal radiotherapy and then I will be CURED!!!!!!!!

If it's all right with all of you, I will continue with the weekly updates as my treatment progresses. My first treatment starts next Thursday which gives me time to recover from today's little op so I will let you know how it goes.

Also I have realized that a lot of my female friends and family (that means you Melanie & Alison) haven't had a smear test done in quite a while—here in Canada you are expected to have one every year and I would feel a lot better if you didn't have to go through what I am going through right now.

Please take this request in the good faith in which I have sent it and be thankful that this is all I am requesting—if my hair falls out, I might be asking for your hair cuttings to stick on my head!!!!!

Anyway, bye for now

Lots of love Louise xxxxx

As odd as it sounds, I was devastated when I was told that I would not be having a hysterectomy. Even though I was terrified at the thought of having to have an operation, I think that I just wanted the cancer to be cut out, I felt like I wouldn't be sure that the cancer would be gone if it wasn't cut away. In hindsight, the treatment that I was given was totally the best option and I am thankful that I didn't have to endure an operation on top of everything else.

Subject: Platinum
Date: Saturday, September 17, 2005

Some of you already know this story which actually makes it funnier!

Way back in the dark ages when Martin & I became a couple I commented one day to my new beau that I could only wear platinum and that silver, gold and white gold irritated my skin!!!!!!!!

Oh how those words have come back to haunt me—my chemotherapy drug is called Cisplatin, the main ingredient being PLATINUM!!!!!

So I guess I really will be a platinum girl now both inside and out!!

I am just reading up on the side effects now and will fill you all in later

Love Louise xx

Subject: cancer week 4 & half
Date: Thursday, September 22, 2005

Treatment day arrives! It is 7am and freezing cold today (currently 1 degree) I feel fairly ok about my appointment today not that I really have any choice!!! I am actually quite glad that the treatment can get under way; waiting around for it to start is horrible.

We have all had a good week; we took mum to the Columbia Icefield and went on the glacier which she was very impressed with, we sang along to Neil Diamond all the way home (a four hour drive) much to Martin's horror!

Martin has started a reflexology course at Calgary University on Friday nights. When he was recovering from his own cancer, reflexology was used as a part of his healing and it really worked for him. We got looking on the internet and the course that Martin wanted to do started last Friday. So now I will get treatments from him all the time which will definitely help with my recovery.

We finally found out who Tom Baker was (thanks to all the Brits who pointed out that Tom Baker was the original Dr Who!) he was a local teacher who throughout his life, raised both money and awareness for cancer research. In 1981 he was rewarded when the new cancer hospital in Calgary was named the Tom Baker Cancer Centre.

The hospital runs a lottery every year in order to raise money, you can buy tickets for $50 and win cars & cash I am not sure if you have to be an Alberta resident to buy a ticket but if you are interested have a look at www.cashandcarslottery.ca

That's about it for now, enjoy the pictures and I will e-mail again after my hospital visit today,

Louise xx

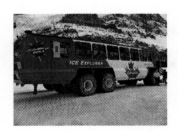

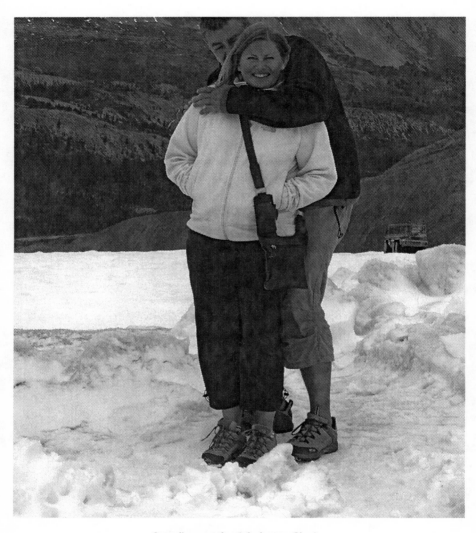

Standing on the Athabasca Glacier

Subject: treatment day 1
Date: Thursday, September 22, 2005

For the first time since my diagnosis, I totally underestimated my appointment today!

I have been feeling great all week and wasn't particularly nervous about today's appointment but as we walked towards the hospital, my feet felt really heavy and I struggled to force myself to go through the door. As we got inside there were some patients waiting for their lifts home and as soon as I saw a man with no legs and a woman with no hair, I got so upset that I just wanted to leave.

I met with my team of specialists (I thought to get my first dose of radiation!) headed now by a Dr Corinne Doll.

I had yet another internal exam (I am beginning to wonder if there is anyone left at the hospital who hasn't seen me naked!!) and then had a 2 hour talk about exactly what is going to happen to me during and after my treatment. I have been booked into a chemo training lecture tomorrow and a plan is being made of my body on computer (they can do wonders with airbrushing maybe I can request that my body plan is thinner!!!)

I have to have another scan on Monday which will determine exactly where the radiation fields will be and will help the doctors to plan my treatment. They will be able to determine how much radiation that I am going to get and then they go ahead and start the treatment.

I will NOT lose my hair on my head although it could thin by up to 50%.

I will lose hair on my legs—hoorah!

I will be infertile—I am sure you all know me well enough to know that this is a good thing!

My periods will stop forever—yipeeeeee think of the money I will save!!!!!

My menopause will start—not good news, risk of osteoporosis and lots of hot flushes!

One other symptom is that the radiation causes the vagina to close slightly and the doctor said the best thing to do to prevent this from happening was to have regular sex! Martin's memory of this conversation however is the doctor said "you have to have sex every day"!

Once the radiation and chemotherapy has been completed (6 weeks) I have a week off and then I have a two day stay in hospital for internal radiation. The internal bit happens twice on two consecutive weeks but I can't explain to you all at the moment what happens because it is a bit gruesome and talking about it makes me feel faint!

Over all the news is very good although going through your menopause at 35 is obviously not great in terms of bone health mainly!

The statistics for my survival, assuming I respond as expected to the treatment, are excellent and this should hopefully be my one and only brush with cancer.

I have to stay away from as many people as I can while I am being treated, particularly children, to avoid any risk of infection and the doctor hopes that any side effects that I do get should be minimal because I have no internal scar tissue (have never been pregnant, not had appendix out etc). The radiation causes scar tissue which in turn causes side effects so as I am otherwise fit and healthy all I should suffer from is acute tiredness and nausea for which I can take tablets.

Thank you Kim, Jamie, Daniel, Tracie, Trudi and Laura for the flowers, they are beautiful. I will sign off now as I have a date with a rather handsome reflexologist!

Louise xxx

At the time of my diagnosis, I didn't want to know too much about my cancer. Although the nurses told me lots of things I really didn't need to know, Dr Doll was very good, only telling me what was absolutely necessary. I had no clue with regards to the stage or size of my cancer and didn't want to know anything about my chances of survival. I really feel that keeping myself in the dark so to speak, was key to keeping a positive mindset.

I was very surprised when, in helping to research this book, Dr Doll supplied the following statistics. When reading them, I am even more convinced that we did the right thing and that sometimes too much information can be damaging.

My actual cancer diagnosis was FIGO (clinical stage) IIB, with left parametrial extension.

Survival statistics: roughly 75% 5-year overall survival (the chance of being alive at 5 years)

70% disease-free survival (the chance of being alive without disease at 5 years).

Subject: Treatment day 1—for real this time!
Date: Monday, September 26, 2005

Hi everyone,

Another long day over we have been at the hospital today for 7 hours!!!! My treatment planning has been done and I have 3 new tattoos, one on my tummy and one on the side of each thigh. I was hoping to get another tattoo anyway and now I have 4 in total! I have also got 3 huge crosses drawn on me with black marker—very attractive! The tattoos didn't hurt nearly as much as when I had the sun on my foot done, I asked the girl if she could do a dolphin, a dragon and a fish but she said she could only draw circles!

The planning of the radiation fields was straight forward (I am sure its quite complicated from the doctors point of view!) I had to lay naked from the waist down, on a narrow bed. A small metal ball bearing was taped to the entrance of my vagina (so it would show up on the scan) then I had to stay very still while the bed moved through an x-ray machine. The tattoos were placed very precisely on my body to ensure that the radiation beams hit the right spot every time.

We took a packed lunch with us as we had to hang around for a couple of hours between appointments and enjoyed the autumn sunshine in the overflow car park.

Treat number 2 for today was a chemotherapy lecture. It was held in an auditorium and there were about 7 cancer patients and their families. Unfortunately the whole thing really freaked me out. They give you so much information that your head feels like it will explode and most of the stuff that they tell you is not relevant as we are obviously all individuals with different types of cancer. We had a tour of the chemo suite, the place was very sterile and even though I have been told, more than once, that I am going to survive this, I couldn't help but notice all of the patients in the room receiving treatment were bald and looked really sick. I was given my list of appointments today, the list of 35 separate visits seems endless and I cried.

I met with Dr Doll and asked a few more questions mostly about the menopause—she has asked that during my periods I should not use tampons anymore because of the risk of excess bleeding so on top of everything else I now have a bloody great mattress thing wedged between my legs!!!! Roll on the menopause!

I am having my first chemo treatment on Tuesday next week at 8am. The nurse has said that the side effects won't kick in for about a week (I hope the sickness doesn't start at all—the anti nausea drugs are $40 each tablet, 3 tablets a day adding that up when you aren't earning anything is scary in fact it makes you feel sick so we won't think about that any more) although my treatment is covered under Alberta health care, they don't pay for drugs!

Will sign off now as I feel very tired and Martin is going to try out the foot massage on me that he learned this week at university.

Will be in touch,

Louise xx

Subject: Cancer week 5 and half.
Date: Wednesday, September 28, 2005

I was having a good day today and then it changed drastically so I thought I would moan to everyone and see if it made me feel better!

I have been having some bad lower back pains which are a symptom of my cancer, and because the pain is fairly constant it is starting to get me down.

The radiation nurse has said that after the first week of treatment I should feel really good but the chemo nurse said that the chemo side effects will kick after the first week! All of the side effects for the 2 treatments seem to conflict—radiation gives you diarrhea and chemotherapy makes you constipated, the radio will stop the stomach & back pain while the chemo will make you vomit! I really just don't know what to expect. It is a shame that they give you so much information because now that I know all of the possible side effects, I am waiting for them to happen—I wonder if that would be so if you weren't told about potential problems and just dealt with symptoms if they arose?

I had a good chat with Jo today (my friend who is moving to New Zealand) and we have been out walking in Fish Creek park, I have to walk every day as it will help me to keep fit during my chemo, the weather has been nice but is definitely getting colder in the mornings now, so all in all no reason to feel down in the dumps!

One thing that did cheer me up—we went to the 7/11 store and bought Cadburys thin chocolate bars (Cadburys animal bars in the UK) my favorite!!!!! They have recently gone on sale in Canada so things aren't all bad!

We bought a pumpkin yesterday and had a bit of a cook off! We made pumpkin and sweet corn soup which was delicious, pumpkin lasagna which was disgusting and flavorless, we threw the lot away, and then we toasted the seeds which are apparently very good for you and ate them all!

Martin has just finished a reflexology treatment on me and my back is feeling a lot better, I just can't seem to settle today, I know I am rambling on in this e-mail but I can't be bothered to re do it now.

I am getting a bit nervous about my first chemo treatment on Tuesday, I keep looking at the list of appointments that the hospital gave me (2 pages long) the chemo is given via an intravenous drip into the back of my hand—I will get Martin to take a picture of me having it then you can see the massive chairs that you have to sit in!!!! It will take about 3 or 4 hours to go in so I hope I get the chair with the nice views of the Bow River. Martin is allowed to sit with me so it shouldn't be too bad, I might sneak the scrabble game in my bag and make him play that with me.

I must be boring you all by now, I am boring myself, so I am going to go and empty the dishwasher, that's if Martin hasn't done it already! I don't seem to have done anything for myself for ages; maybe I'll go and paint my fingernails!

Louise x

Subject: Chemo day 1
Date: Tuesday, October 04, 2005

I really don't know where to start—we woke at 6am this morning and I didn't feel nervous to the same extent as before, I actually felt quite excited to be getting started.

We got to the hospital 15 minutes early and on the journey there it crossed my mind that maybe I should tie back my hair or even wear a hat in case the sight of my hair made anyone feel bad! I know it sounds nuts but I really felt I might offend the people who had lost their hair.

In the waiting room it became very apparent that people with no hair really don't care—I was amazed that no one seemed to make any effort with their hats or head coverings at all and I would like to think that should I lose my hair (v. small chance of that happening) I would choose a spectacular hat and make sure I looked pretty darned good!

Still the thought of my potential new headwear gave us something to giggle at aside from the woman who sat talking to the goldfish, Martin nick named her Wanda! She actually turned out to be very nice, a long distance runner with lung cancer. We took turns in peeing for four hours—more on that later!

The nurses were very kind and chatted about nothing in particular whilst setting up my iv. I lay on a comfy bed with my book, 2 oatmeal bars, 2 cookies, 2 cups of tea and 2 litres of water and Martin of course! Martin was most impressed when he realized that the TV worked and he could catch up on the bike racing. He made a passing comment about whether the remote control worked every television and before I could stop him he aimed the control at a TV in a cubicle on the far side of the room and we watched in horror as the channel changed from a calm holiday program to Speed TV super bike racing!!!!!! He swears that he never dreamt the control would work but I couldn't stop laughing especially as he felt so bad—not bad enough to own up though!

I had 5 different bags of fluid over four hours and didn't feel a thing, oh I didn't get a window bed either, probably just as well as it was very sunny and we wouldn't have been able to see the television!

Wanda, aka Constance, my new fish loving friend, stopped by on her very regular visits to the bathroom and said she could tell it was my first time as I looked scared in the waiting room (and there's me thinking I was being brave!) she chatted about her cancer and asked about mine, she was on her fifth cycle of chemo and looked remarkably well. The fluid starts to kick in after half an hour and from then on you are up and down to the bathroom every five minutes. You also have to drink a lot of water as the chemo can do serious damage to your kidneys so you need to flush it through.

I was so impressed with the nurses and the volunteers who make the tea and cookies, next time I won't be worried at all.

We finished in the chemo suite at about 1pm and walked around outside to get some air—we bought a sandwich in a deli and got totally ripped off but I'll fill you in on that one later, if I get on my soap box now I'll be typing all night!

Back to hospital for radiation, I had some more maps drawn on me which I mustn't wash off so my belly resembles a football pitch with huge crosses at either end for goals and I am not allowed to use bubble bath or any perfumed products as I will get a sunburn mark the whole way around my pelvic area—definitely must buy some Bridget Jones knickers to avoid any rubbing!!!!

Two different men were working in the radiation lab today bringing my total of hospital staff seeing me naked to about 40!!!! I have absolutely no dignity left, in fact when Constance asked me about my cancer today I very nearly showed her!

Finally we arrived home today at about 4.30pm very tired but relieved. I feel so positive now that treatment is under way. I am taking a multi vitamin every day and drinking pomegranate juice by the gallon—thanks to mum and John Hooper for the tip (apparently it is the new anti cancer super food in the UK).

Thank you Melanie and Jason for the Sudoku books they will come in handy especially on chemo days and on Friday nights when Martin is at university.

Thank you all for your lovely e-mails—I really do appreciate the time you take to write and I am sorry that I don't always respond to every one individually.

Lots of love Louise xxx

The sandwich story: We didn't want to eat in the hospital so decided to visit the deli that was near the hospital. Bear in mind that this deli is the only non—fast food, non—greasy food option in the hospital vicinity, and probably gets most of its business from hospital staff and patients, we ordered two egg salad sandwiches to take away. The bill was $21! That was an awful lot of money for 2 sandwiches in Calgary, so we were expecting them to be huge, fresh and tasty.

We took our lunch to a sunny, grassy spot to eat and when we unwrapped the bag, mouths watering, what a shock—nasty, day old, cardboard bread, rubber eggs with too much mayonnaise and not enough egg and two slices of carrot which we guessed was supposed to be the salad.

Neither one of us had the energy to return to the shop nor would we ever eat there again, on subsequent visits we took a packed lunch with us.

Subject: chemo week 2
Date: Monday, October 10, 2005

I can't believe Tuesday has arrived again, once this chemo is over I only have 4 more to go!

This last week has been very odd to say the least, I really didn't know what to expect after my treatment last week so was very nervous when I got home. It's quite a long day because I still have to have the radiotherapy as well so Tuesday we are in hospital pretty much all day.

The nurses gave me 24 different anti nausea drugs to take over the 3 days following chemo, they couldn't categorically say that the drugs would definitely stop the sickness, as apparently they don't always work for everyone, and I really feel that I am having enough crap put into my body at the moment so I decided not to take them! Over all it was a good decision although I did get some waves of nausea, the biggest problem was waiting for something to happen—when we went to hospital on the Wednesday, I had to see my doctor and I told her that I hadn't taken the drugs, she looked at me like I was completely mad and said she thought I should take them as soon as I got home! (I didn't bother).

I decided that I would take each day hour by hour, so I would get up at 8am and tell myself that I don't need the tablets right away, I will see how I feel at 9am and take them at that time if necessary. Then at 9am I would be fine and think I will have some breakfast and see how I feel at 10am. I worked through 3 or 4 days using this pattern until I decided that I was clearly going to be fine without the anti nausea tablets.

The biggest problem that has occurred so far is a severely heightened sense of smell. We went out for a walk on Thursday and passed a woman coming out of her house who was wearing perfume. I had to run away as quickly as I could as I thought I was going to throw up on her front lawn!

I had real trouble eating on Tuesday, Wednesday, Thursday and Friday, the smell of anything cooking made me feel sick and when I did eat it was taking ages as I had to chew really slowly so the food stayed down, on Saturday however my appetite returned with a vengeance! I had some chocolate in the fridge that had survived days untouched (very unusual in our house) because the smell of it turned my stomach, since Saturday I have eaten 2 twirl bars, 8 Cadbury thins, 3 bananas, 2 oranges, 1 large tin of peaches, 10 slices of toast and butter, 1 fried egg, 3 bran muffins, 2 homemade burgers, 1 tin spaghetti hoops, 2 chicken breasts, cauliflower, broccoli, carrots and yams, 3 homemade brownies and an enormous thanksgiving turkey dinner! Oh and I just had an egg sandwich!

I am still quite anxious when it gets to bed time; Martin thinks it may have something to do with the thought of surviving 12 hours through the night without food!

The absolute worst side effect has been emotionally. I feel like a blob of meat going to be micro waved every day; you loose all dignity and self confidence as well. Most of you already know that I have never had much of a problem in the confidence department (which maybe makes this worse?) but I have had a couple of panic attacks and don't seem able to make the smallest of decisions. In the beginning, Martin was doing everything for me and I really struggled with that but now I happily sit there and let him do everything just so that I don't have to think! Every time the phone goes, I panic in case I have to talk about the cancer I know it is ridiculous and I don't feel like it all of the time but mostly I just feel useless!

Not much has happened on the hair front, I did stop myself yesterday as I was about to complain that my hair was flyaway and driving me mad—only a couple of weeks ago I was terrified that I would lose it all. It definitely is drying out so I may get it cut shorter just to keep it looking nice. Looking forward to leg hair loss which should happen this week some time, not looking forward to pubic hair loss, I am not sure why it just seems weird!

The radiotherapists draw on my tummy every day so I look a bit like a car crash victim naked, my skin generally feels odd and I still feel very squeamish looking at myself in the mirror even though there is nothing but a few drawings to look at, I can't touch my body either, nothing hurts but I just feel weird and a bit goose bumpy.

Martin watched one of my radiotherapy treatments last week and was very impressed with the laser equipment. After he fiddled with the TV remote in the chemo suite, I made it clear he wasn't to touch any buttons while I was being zapped—can you imagine the damage he could do?

Each day my appointment for my radiotherapy is only 10 minutes long, most of that time is spent getting me lined up on the bed correctly—I have to lie on a grid that is placed on a bed. The area receiving the radiation is then exposed (naked again I hear you cry!) and I have to keep very still which is surprisingly difficult especially as I also have to have a full bladder. Once the technicians have set me in the right place, they leave the room but can still see me and speak to me. The bed is raised a fair way off the ground and the radiation machine moves into position.

The machine is very noisy, it moves to three different positions, zapping its beam into me as it moves around my body. The zapping part only lasts for about 2 minutes and is completely painless.

Thanks Elaine and Steve for the flowers they are lovely and to Andrea and Clint for the thanksgiving invite (sorry we couldn't come but I just have to be reclusive at the moment).

I am off to bed now—I have been sleeping about 13 hours a night and I have an early appointment tomorrow—9.15am chemotherapy and 2.30pm radiotherapy.

Fingers crossed that I am as well this week as I was last week,

Lots of love Louise xxx

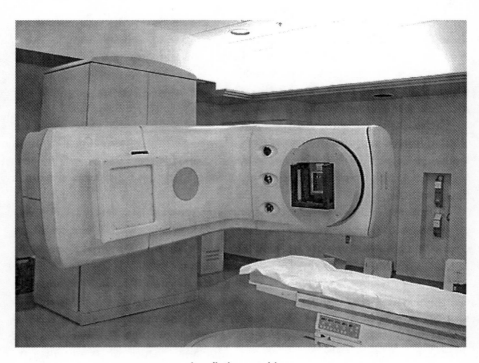

A radiation machine.

Subject: cancer—top of the class!
Date: Wednesday, October 12, 2005

Well its 4am and I am wide awake!

Yesterday's chemo went really well. I have to be weighed on a Tuesday and I was the only patient to gain weight—2lb hoorah (well a bit embarrassing actually) I am clearly on the way to being the fattest cancer patient ever! The doctors seemed very pleased with me so felt a tiny bit smug!

When you get the chemo, the iv pumps 4 litres of fluid (drugs, medication and saline) onto your body and you are told to drink as much as you physically can on top of that to flush everything through. I usually aim to drink a litre and a half in hospital, a litre on the way home and a further 2 litres throughout the rest of the day. So on our return home yesterday, I insisted that we complete our daily walk—do you know where I am going with this yet?

On good days we walk through Fish Creek Park but yesterday we just walked around the block which used to take 40 minutes and now takes closer to an hour! I peed twice before we set off and 2 blocks from home had to sprint to the 7-11 store to go again! I'll be fine now I insisted to Martin who was keen to go home! Famous last words!

Four blocks from the 7-11 and 5 from home the urge to pee hit again oh my god—I was so desperate I even knocked on a strangers door but no one was home, I contemplated sitting on the grass verge and just going there but managed to half walk half run until I got half a block from home and I could see the open garage door (Martin ran on ahead to open the door) when I started to pee myself!

Thankfully I made it into the garage before things got too embarrassing but oh my god what a horrible experience, I peed in a bucket in the garage because I could hold it no more! We completed the walk in 25 minutes though!

Obviously the moral of this story is—what goes in must come out!

Anyway take care and don't laugh too hard at my expense

Louise xxx

Subject: 3.20 am!
Date: Saturday, October 15, 2005

Hi everyone,

It's the middle of the night and once again I am wide awake! The last week has been great, my chemo went well on Tuesday and I still feel relatively healthy! I have not been sick at all and am still not taking my sickness drugs. I am however feeling very tired most of the time and get extremely breathless as the day goes on—this is apparently normal and expected so nothing to worry about!

The radiation team had to re measure my cancer yesterday which is excellent news as it means that the treatment is working and the tumor is shrinking already!

I am crossing off appointments daily from my schedule and am now exactly half way down the first page—I know it seems like a small thing but marking the days off helps me to feel positive.

My last chemo is on November 10th and after that I just have to have two overnight stays in hospital for the internal radiation and then I will be done! Roll on December then I can get back to normality!

I have to say that it seems quite apparent from our daily visits to hospital that the majority of cancer patients that seem to be thriving are the ones who aren't working as they receive treatment. It is unfortunate that lots of people don't have the luxury of taking the time to recover but how you would get through this hell and hold down a job is way beyond me!

I am still pretty paranoid about catching infections and now have some lovely blue masks to wear whenever I am out and about! When I went to radiation yesterday, the doctor said I had to "air the area" more so now I have to walk around butt naked at home as well as in hospital—not a sight for the faint hearted!!!!

My appetite hasn't calmed down at all and I have been getting very odd cravings! I can't seem to each any sweet stuff any more, it just doesn't taste right but I have eaten lots of eggs and broccoli. I am also desperate to get my hands on some Heinz salad cream—we can't find it here although I know Kim is on the look out for the little sachets for me!

My hair hasn't thinned much but looks very dry and lifeless at the moment—Steve I'd be grateful for any tips! I have given up counting the hairs that end up it my hairbrush, it seemed a fruitless task anyway and I don't look that different at the moment. No other hair loss to report at the moment, rest assured you'll be the first to know!

My skin is fairing quite well and I am trying to drink at least 3 litres of water every day to flush out the toxins from the chemo, the radiation area is dry but not sore at all and I have to use Johnson's baby powder every day after a bath.

Our visas have been renewed for another year—still can't believe that we haven't received our permanent ones yet although the Calgary Herald ran a story last week saying that there were approximately 700,000 outstanding applications waiting in immigration departments around the world to be processed! Unfortunately London is one of the biggest administration centers for this backlog and accepts applications not only from England but from many other countries around the world and there are apparently only 3 immigration officers working at Canada House in London who are qualified to sign off paperwork!

Well I am going to try and go back to sleep for a while, have a good weekend

Louise xxxx

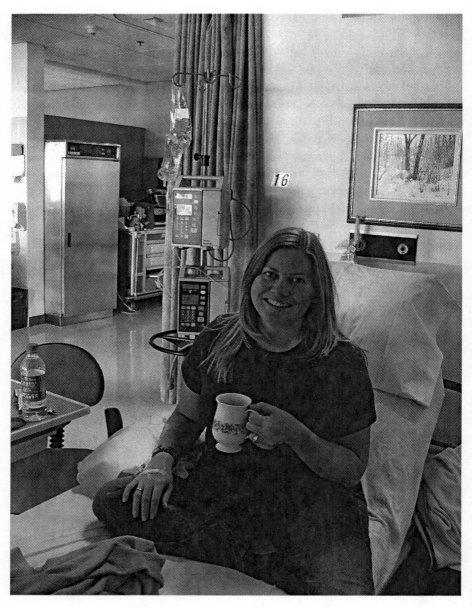

Me having chemo and a cuppa!

Subject: Chemo week 3
Date: Tuesday, October 18, 2005

Hi guys,

Well I made it to the half way point and the psychological effect that has is pretty overwhelming! I feel very tired tonight and also a bit emotional. The chemo went very well today and we had a bit of a laugh with the nurses. One poor lady was having her 2nd treatment and they couldn't find a useable vein, 5 nurses tried to locate a vein and the whole ward fell about laughing when Martin offered assistance and volunteered to do it for them! We were trying to work out what letters Martin will have after his name when is becomes a qualified reflexologist—the best one I could come up with was Martin Lampard P.R.A.T—practitioner of reflexology applied techniques. Let me know if you can think of anything better!

Radiotherapy is becoming very tiring and I really look forward to Fridays when I know I have the weekend off, but by this Friday I shall be half way through that as well!

My food cravings have taken a bizarre turn this week, peanut butter has featured quite highly as have brussel sprouts! I have upped my liquid intake again this week and now try to down at least 4 litres of fluids every day (and that's not in alcohol before anyone comments!). Water really seems to be a really positive factor as far as keeping the nausea at bay and I am still not taking my sickness drugs by the way.

My weeks now fall into a very definite pattern of physical as well as emotional side effects, on Monday evenings; I get that feeling of dread in the pit of my stomach because the week for me feels like it starts on a Tuesday.

Tuesdays—all day in hospital, very tired and a bit down. Not much appetite, pee loads!

Wednesdays—waves of nausea, lethargic, good mental attitude, no appetite.

Thursdays—energized, feel generally better not much nausea or appetite. Normally cry a bit!

Fridays—extra exercise today, eat better feel great again but constipated—take herbal laxative!!!

Saturday, Sunday, Monday—eat everything in sight feel fantastic, lots more energy, glad another week is over.

And that is the sum of my very dull life! Basically the weekends are great and this whole experience so far isn't as bad as I was expecting—note that none of my days are taken up with anything that could be remotely described as a chore—Martin has turned into a super human wife and doesn't sit still for one minute from the moment he wakes up!

That's all for this week, I am off to bed!

Louise x

Subject: blood tests!
Date: Friday, October 21, 2005

Hi all,

I know it's not my usual day to write but I wanted to give you all a quick update. My visit with my oncologist this week went very well and she was both pleased and very surprised to tell me that my white blood cell count (the cells that take care of my immune system) is still normal!

This is quite an unusual turn of events as most normal people would be severely immuno-compromised by now. But fantastic for me as it means my body is doing a great job of fighting and at present I still have good immunity to coughs & colds etc.

Anyway, I just wanted to say thank you to my mum and dad for my strong constitution, thanks to Martin for looking after me so well and feeding me all the right things and thanks to you all for keeping my spirits high.

Have a good weekend,

Louise xxx

Subject: chemo week 4
Date: Tuesday, October 25, 2005

We just got home from another long hospital visit and I am very tired so forgive my typing errors!

Today's chemo went very well again although the ward were short staffed so it makes the day longer as the nurses don't get to change your iv bags as quickly as they normally would! There were 3 nurses training to insert iv's today and they were using a dummy arm, Martin has volunteered his veins for next weeks training session so that should be fun to watch! In fact I might even take the camera with me if I remember.

It is very comical to see people as they enter the chemo suite, although most of us patients don't know each other; we all go through a very similar routine. Almost everyone brings a spouse or friend, a packed lunch, chocolate, a book, a couple of bottles of water and something to donate to the ward (a hat, magazine, flowers etc) I hadn't taken a lot of notice until now but it made me smile today watching other people all unconsciously doing the same thing!

The radiation machine broke today so we had a bit of a wait for the maintenance crew to come and fix it, not a problem under normal circumstances but I have to have a full bladder during my treatment so the big question was to pee or not to pee! Luckily it only took 10 minutes to fix!

I still am not suffering any major side effects, my skin is dry but hasn't burnt yet and my hair is thinner but not really noticeable to anyone but me. Thankfully my appetite has calmed down and I managed to lose 3 pounds this week. I am still eating really well just not to the same extremes as before!

This week's cravings have been for Kellogg's crunchy nut cornflakes and cheese! Martin went to Safeway to buy me the cereal but they don't have it here, they have something called honey crunch which looked the same but tasted different, I ate it anyway and they craving passed. I have some salad cream winging its way from the UK and the thought of it is making my mouth water!

Thanks to Aunty Trudy for the lovely letter you sent. Well done James & Jo on selling your house—one step closer to NZ!

Hope you all have a good week

Love Louise xx

Subject: chemo week 5
Date: Wednesday, November 02, 2005

Hi everyone,

Well week 5 of chemo out of the way—what can I say?

This last week has not been great for feeling sick, Wednesday and Thursday I had nausea pretty much the whole time which isn't pleasant. My appetite has suffered because of it and although I still have cravings for certain foods, I haven't hit my previous highs of food intake! My weight is stable though so that's good.

My doctor examined my cancer on Wednesday and was quite surprised at how much it has shrunk—the staff are beginning to treat me like a medical marvel, my white blood counts are still normal!!!!

We had a great time in the radiation unit on Halloween, all the staff dressed up and decorated the unit and the children (patients and kids of patients) wandered about trick or treating. The staff had a pumpkin carving contest and were cheered on by the patients.

I have stopped my daily walking, partly due to lethargy and partly due to the SNOW!!! Yes we have snow once again. Actually it only just snowed last night so I can't really blame my laziness on the weather.

My senses have calmed down a bit, now I am only really affected by lots of noise or really strong scent. I haven't got any aches or pains at all and my pubic hair has only just started to fall out—a very weird experience, and one I wouldn't recommend! My sister sent me some excellent hair conditioner—thanks Melanie—as my hair is really looking rough now, I would definitely pass as trailer trash! If the conditioner doesn't work, I am going to get my hair cut shorter and just wear lots of hats!

We are both growing tired of the daily runs to hospital—I think the truck knows its own way there now although it has been emotionally uplifting this week to be discussing the end of my treatment, my hospital dates have been booked for my internal radiation Nov 22nd–24th and Nov 29-Dec 1st. I will be told six weeks after that if the cancer has gone and I have the all clear. Whilst I am in hospital, I will be radioactive for 24 hours so Martin can't be with me, they do however give me a phone in my room so I will get a couple of long distance phone cards and call some of you to take my mind off things!

My last chemo is on Tuesday and my last regular radiation is on Thursday next week then I have a week off to let my cervix recover before the final onslaught. My menopause has started and I am experiencing hot flushes every now and then! I have to see my original oncologist to discuss HRT, I don't think he will be surprised to find out that I want to do this naturally and not have tablets!

Well I have only cried once this week and they were tears of relief after yesterday's chemo. I had a beautiful card yesterday from Daniel with lovely Sharks tale stickers on it (Daniel is 5 years old) so thank you Daniel. Thanks Melanie for the hair stuff.

Lots of love

Louise xxxxx

Subject: chemo week 6.
Date: Wednesday, November 09, 2005

Hi everyone,

Hope you have all had a good week, I really don't know where to start this week so I think I will just go day by day starting with last Wednesday.

Wednesday November 2nd

We had our appointment with Dr Doll today and her nurse discussed with us the internal treatment that I will be getting, she showed us photo's which looked pretty horrific but I think that boredom will be my biggest problem as I will have to lay perfectly still for 24 hours and am not allowed visitors! Then I got a present … a vaginal dilator! I am sorry to share all the gory details but I know that some people reading this are going through the same as me and hopefully this may take away the element of surprise! Anyway, this plastic candle looking object has to be inserted and wiggled for 10 minutes, 3 times a week! It is basically to keep the cervix area open for future doctor's examinations but still rather unpleasant!

Thursday November 3rd

I felt sick all day and very tired, I haven't done any exercise for days and am finding it a huge effort just to walk up the stairs. Martin pulled a muscle in his shoulder and is in quite a bit of pain. My radiation team informed us today that I have only 2 treatments next week and not four as scheduled, I cried but not sure why as I should be happy! I am nervous of the treatment finishing.

Friday November 4th

Bad day again today, I was actually sick this morning for the first time and then suffered nausea all day, I haven't eaten much this week and can't wait for bed time as Saturday's are usually good days. The nurse rang to say my white blood count was too low and my chemo won't be done on Tuesday unless it improves, they will put the chemo off for a week—very upset, I just want this to be over.

Saturday November 5th

Bonfire night in England—I used to love watching the fireworks and I got up feeling homesick until I spoke to my mum who informed us that it had rained all day which doesn't bode well for an enjoyable Guy Fawkes Night. I feel better and not sick today, I am getting excited now about my last chemo and hope that a blood test on Monday shows improvement in my blood count. Martin feels better so is going to do lots of work on my foot spleen reflex as this can help to produce masses of white blood cells—fingers crossed.

Sunday November 6th

More reflexology today, I am feeling really good today, it snowed last night and we walked this morning in the park near our house. I felt really proud of myself when we got home although I slept for 2 hours as I was exhausted!

Monday November 7th

Radiation and blood test today—all is well and my chemo can go ahead tomorrow as planned. We are both looking forward to a lay in on Wednesday; the daily hospital visits have become a real chore. I joked with the team today that as I had had no real side effects of the treatment, I was going to get them all in one go tomorrow and would probably arrive for my appointment near death and in a wheel chair! How those words came back to haunt me.

Tuesday November 8th

I feel very nervous for some reason today and also quite tearful. I was up most of the night as the diarrhea seems to have started. I sat next to a friend, Wendy, today who has breast cancer; it was also her last treatment today so we chatted about how great we were feeling and both ended up crying! Her husband is also called Martin but he calls himself Marty and insists on calling my Martin the same except with his accent he pronounced it 'Mardy' and it made me laugh. Wendy finished her chemo before me so she hugged us both as she left and promised to stay in touch.

My chemo nurses today are Robbi and Carleen and it seems quite fitting that they gave me my first treatment and are here to share my last.

The chemo started to run through the iv as usual and just before it was half way through, I started to cough. Just a tickle at first and then it got worse, my chest went red and Martin was trying to get me to sip water. Robbi came to check on me just as my face started to swell! I was having an allergic reaction to the chemo. They unhooked me immediately and started pumping drugs through my iv, by now I was surrounded by nurses and doctors and I was terrified. My face and torso were covered in bright red welts and my blood pressure was reading 165/123 and rising. The crash team were put on standby and a lady came to do an ECG which lets face was not going to be normal under the circumstances! Also I have a small heart valve defect that causes no problem other than it gives dodgy ECG readings so got everyone in a panic! Martin was trying to explain this to the doctor as the drugs that I had been given kicked in and we all started to relax. A nurse took me to the bathroom and when I saw myself in the mirror I could see why Martin looked so scared.

I lay covered in cold cloths while the doctors decided what to do with me. After about an hour, the redness started to fade and my face looked near normal again. Robbi advised that I wouldn't be having the rest of my chemo and that it will have no detrimental effect on the outcome of my treatment. I was sent down to radiation in a wheelchair and told to go back to chemo afterwards for another ECG. The radiation went smoothly and it was sad saying goodbye to John, Salima and Kleve aka Theresa.[2]

They assured me that they would never see me again and that I had been a model patient.

Back to chemo, the ECG was done and I was thoroughly checked out. My iv was removed and we said a teary goodbye to the nurses.

I can't celebrate with alcohol at the moment so we drove to Dairy Queen and I had a chocolate brownie explosion. It was huge, delicious, really fattening and I ate every last bit!!!

---

2.   I was first introduced to Kleve when I was shown around the radiation unit. I waited in a private room on my own for a radiation technician to explain what would happen to me during my treatment. Kleve was the designated technician—he shook my hand and said "Hi I'm Kleve but most people call me Theresa" I shook his hand and said hello, completely ignoring his joke remark about his name—clearly I was so stressed out, it didn't even register in my brain that he was trying to be funny to relax me!

Wednesday November 9th 5am

Wide awake, feeling great and writing an e-mail to all of my friends.

Lots of love

Louise xxxxx

ps Mum, I really am fine now so don't ring me until later because Martin is obviously still asleep!

Subject: cancer week 12 and half
Date: Wednesday, November 16, 2005

Hi everyone,

Just a short e-mail this week as nothing much to report. After last weeks drama I recovered quite quickly and have been feeling better every day.

I had a doctor's check up today and she is very pleased with my progress. She explained again what will happen when I am admitted to the ward next Tuesday for my Brachytherapy, it doesn't sound pleasant but I don't have a choice! My e-mail next week will not be until Friday so I can let you know what it was like.

One thing that does bug me is both the doctor and the nurse say that this next procedure is nothing more than uncomfortable and that I will feel a bit like a stuffed turkey! I really wanted to say "how the hell do you know"? I know that they do this procedure quite regularly but they have never personally been 'stuffed' with 3 metal tubes, 3 feet of gauze and had their flaps sewn together!

Maybe I am just being over sensitive!

Martin was actually quite concerned because all through my treatment I have made him do everything with me (he actually took laxatives when I had to take them) He is worried that he doesn't have space for 3 tubes and packing and what on earth will the doctor stitch together!

That's it for this week,

Love Louise xx

Brachytherapy, also known as sealed source radiotherapy or endocuriether-apy, is a form of radiotherapy where a radioactive source is placed inside or next to the area requiring treatment.

Intracavitary brachytherapy places the sources inside a pre-existing body cavity. The most common applications of this method are gynaecological in nature.

Remote Afterloading Machines

Although manual afterloading reduced exposures, the guiding principle of radiation protection is to keep exposures as low as reasonably achievable (ALARA) given prevailing economic, political and societal factors. The move to reduce exposures even further led to the introduction of *remote afterloading*. This technique relies on the use of hollow tubes which are connected to a safe containing a small radioactive source welded to a wire that is driven out by a stepping motor to predetermined positions to deliver radiation dose.

These machines deliver their treatment remotely. A plan is produced that describes the patterns of the stepping motor (distance and dwell time). The motor is only engaged when all staff have left the shielded room that holds the patient for the duration of the treatment.

This means that the nurse or therapeutic radiographer that administers can leave the room (located either in theatre or ward) and start the treatment outside. Empty catheters are placed into the patient and the 'live' source is entered at a later date. This means that the non-active dummy guides can be repositioned and checked. In other words, the source is not placed into the guides until the positioning is acceptable. The machine then runs a pneumatic drive wire through the catheters and guide wires to check that there are no obstructions and the source can safely run through the course of it. After this the check has been performed the source leaves its secure safe and the treatment begins.

Low Dose Rate (LDR) brachytherapy is a common brachytherapy method. Applicators in the form of catheters are arranged, usually according to the Manchester or Paris system on, or in the patient. A low dose rate source is then driven along the catheters on the end of a wire by a machine while the patient is isolated in a room. The source dwells in a preplanned position for a preset time before stepping forward along the catheter and repeating, to build up the required dose distribution. The advantage of this treatment over implanting radioactive sources directly is that there is lower staff exposure and the source can be more active due to low staff exposure, thus making treatment times quicker.

For my intracavitary brachytherapy, I had three hollow, metal tubes (rather like empty Bic pen tubes but longer) called a full Fletcher-suit inserted into my vagina and then the vagina is stuffed with packing and stitched to hold into place. I would be hooked up to a radiation machine for two courses of twenty four hours each.

Once the correct radiation dose had been given, the packing, stitches and apparatus would be removed and I would go home, returning within seven days for another insertion and the next twenty four hour dose. Dr Doll had explained that I would be unable to move during this procedure in order to protect the apparatus from moving about.

I would be laying, flat on my back with my knees very slightly bent. As you can imagine, that position is especially uncomfortable to be in for any length of time. I was concerned about going to the toilet but the nurses had said that during the insertion operation, a catheter would be started and I would be given drugs as well as a low fibre diet to stop any bowel movements.

Subject: Good news and Bad news!
Date: Wednesday, November 23, 2005

Hi everyone,

Bad news first—I am not in hospital as expected, the procedure had to be stopped as the insertion of the apparatus accidentally punctured my uterus! Details below!!!!! (Don't read if you are squeamish)

Good news—There is no sign of any cancer in my body at all. The ultrasound doctor that saw me today asked me why I was in the cancer centre—he could see nothing wrong with me at all (apart from an extra hole in my womb).

Extra good news—I won a competition in last weeks newspaper, 2 tickets to the ski world championships at Lake Louise and a $50 gas voucher!

My week so far has gone something like this:

Monday pm November 21st

Nervous about tomorrow, mostly worried that I will die under anesthetic. I know that this is a totally irrational fear but I am scared nonetheless.

Tuesday November 22nd

We arrived at the hospital at 5.30pm, I had my weight and blood pressure checked and filled in lots of forms. After an ECG and a chest x-ray we were told that we could leave the hospital as long as we returned by 9pm. We got home at 7pm had an egg sandwich and watched American chopper! I cried through most of the program.

Back at the hospital, I had to change into one of those awful gowns that never do up properly and my nurse came in to give me an enema. Martin said that from the sounds he heard coming from the bathroom, he thought I was trying to escape on a high revving vespa!

Martin left me at midnight and I finally fell asleep about 1.30am. Wide awake at 4am I was very nervous this morning, Martin arrived at 6am and the nurse gave me a blood thinning injection, Heparin (it has left an enormous bruise on my arm!). After my vaginal douche (I won't go into details but at least it didn't hurt) I had to put on thigh length support socks and wait for the porter to take me to theatre. As you can imagine, I was looking superb!

I was sobbing like a baby when I saw my doctor and she reassured me that the pain would be controlled by morphine and she was only inserting the apparatus in holes that were already there (how wrong she was!) so my discomfort would be minimal.

When I opened my eyes in the recovery room, I was pleasantly surprised to feel not much at all, Martin was holding my hand and I saw Dr Doll standing next to me, I was horrified when they told me that they hadn't carried out the insertion and had pushed the probe into my uterus and out the other side!

I had a saline iv running and was sent to the ultrasound dept for further investigation. The technician couldn't get a clear picture from my tummy so I had to have an internal ultrasound—on a normal day this would not be too much of a problem but after half an operation and a stab wound to the uterus need I say more …

I now have a course of antibiotics to stop internal infection to the wound and the doctor will try again next week. They did measure me today using the scan and ultrasound picture so next week they know exactly how far to insert the centre probe.

The doctor apologized and doesn't expect to have any further problems next week; I still have to have both procedures so my treatment will now end in two weeks time.

We got home about 2.30pm today both very tired and me very sore. I am holding on to the positive news that there is no trace of cancer left in me, the doctor who performed the internal ultra sound asked me why I was in a cancer hospital, he couldn't see any sign of anything wrong with me so I hope that the next two weeks fly past.

Love to everyone, Louise xx

During my insertion operation there had been several doctors present. My uterus is posterior and retroverted (tilted towards my back) and unfortunately the doctor given the unenviable task of inserting the apparatus, had used the correct measurements given to them by Dr Doll but hadn't taken into account the tilting of my uterus thus an error was made during the placement.

Fortunately the uterus is a bit like a sponge so any hole made will close almost immediately and in fact, the doctor who carried out the internal ultrasound afterwards couldn't see anything wrong with me when he examined my uterus, also the ultrasound images taken at that time, were subsequently used to ensure that the apparatus was place correctly during the second attempt.

Subject: it's been a long week!
Date: Sunday December 4, 2005

I don't know what to say other than
IT'S OVER IT'S OVER IT'S OVER!!!
Okay, here's how it went ...

Tuesday night November 29th

I checked into hospital at 7.30pm and had an ECG, chest x-ray, blood tests, enema temperature, weight, height and blood pressure then I said goodbye to Martin. He was going to stay the night at the hospital as the weather was so bad but we figured it was best for him to go home and try to get a good nights sleep. I was still very nervous although not as bad as I had been the previous week. My nurse said Martin could be back to see me at 6am and stay with me until the radiation machine was hooked up to me. I didn't sleep well and was already awake when the nurse came to wake me at 5.30am.

Wednesday November 30th

Martin arrived at 6am and I had to do a vaginal douche and have a heparin injection to keep my blood thin. (Unfortunately due to the nature of the injection, you get a huge bruise and now I have had six doses, I look like I've been in a fight—and lost!) I only got tearful as I was wheeled down to the operating theatre, I was half hoping that the procedure would fail again as I knew that my doctor wouldn't try for a third time! I asked to see Dr Doll, I think I just wanted to make sure she was there to insert the apparatus this time, as I hadn't seen her and then don't remember much else until I was in the recovery room.

As I woke up Dr Doll was smiling at me saying that all had gone well and they were exceptionally pleased with the placing of the instruments, she also asked if I thought I could manage to do 48 hours instead of 24 as she was concerned that she could not guarantee placing the equipment so well a second time. Obviously I was overjoyed at the prospect of going through this procedure only once and agreed immediately—then the pain hit me!!!!!!

I saw Martin for a while in recovery then he was sent up to my room to wait for me, I was given 2 injections for the pain but the only lasted about 10 minutes before their effect wore off but was promised morphine as soon as I was in my room.

My room had been transformed into a star trek film set, the equipment that holds the radiation is enormous and very weird looking. Dr Doll arrived within minutes and was keen to get things set up, she attached the tubing from the machine to the metal tubes sticking out of me, I was given a shot of morphine, said goodbye to Martin and then everyone left the room to turn on the machine. I had thought that it would take longer for some reason and felt very alone when everyone left. The nurses were told to communicate with me via an intercom and were only to enter the room when they absolutely had to as the machine had to be switched off every time the door opened. So there I was, radioactive and spaced out on morphine—which incidentally confirmed what I had always thought, I could never take drugs, and the feeling of being out of it was just horrible, in the words of my good friend Clint 'I was just weirded out'.

Earlier that morning, Martin had complained of feeling sick, I felt sick too and we put it down to nerves. However on his way out of the hospital, he couldn't stop vomiting and was really concerned that he had a bug and might have given it to me. He phoned me to let me know to warn the nurses as I was on an immune suppressed ward and also my blood test the night before had shown that my own white blood count was extremely low. The morphine knocked me out for a few hours, I think I phoned my mum but other than that I don't remember much until I vomited! I didn't have time to call the nurse and as I was lying down I threw up all over myself. It seemed to take a long time for the nurses to come and help me; they changed my nightgown but couldn't change the bed so they just covered it over with towels. I washed what I could of my neck, face and shoulders with a face cloth and just prayed that I had missed my hair! I was sick 4 more times so the nurses set up an iv with anti sickness drugs and a glucose/saline drip.

I have never watched so much rubbish on television in all my life and I am thankful that I remembered to take an international phone card in with me. I couldn't eat as I have a lot of mouth ulcers (from the chemo) and also I was worried about eating whilst lying down in case I choked. (Also a bit concerned about having to go to the toilet, I had a catheter for the pee but hadn't counted on staying in bed for 48 hours!)

Wednesday night I slept fairly well on and off but from Thursday morning I was pretty much awake until Friday night! I spoke to lots of friends in England as well as in Canada and watched Everybody loves Raymond a lot on TV.

My room looked like a bomb site, when my meals were brought in; the nurses had to be quick so instead of clearing away my previous meal trays, they just stacked them all over the room, placing the current tray on my bed, table thingy. Consequently, after three or four mealtimes, my room smelt very bad.

I really wished I had taken in some chewing gum as I had a mouth full of ulcers and found it almost impossible to clean my teeth. I didn't eat very much at all, partly because of the ulcers and partly because I was concerned that I would choke as I was eating lying down! I think I would have been better off with those meals in a can so I could have drunk rather than chewed.

The last six hours really dragged, I got very upset on Friday morning and phoned Martin in a bit of a state, I think I was just very tired and wanted it to be over by that stage. Dr Doll came to see me when I had just 2 hours to go, she was really up beat and so pleased with my progress.

1.18pm on Friday the machine switched off. Dr Doll and her colleague came in to unhook me. The nurse gave me some more morphine and the doctor took out the stitches (that was the only bit that hurt) they sprayed the packing with water to loosen it and then unraveled it and took out the metal tubes. Sitting up was traumatic, I felt so dizzy and faint that it took a further 3 hours before I could stand unaided. My hair looked horrendous, the front of my hair was the greasiest it has ever been, I had a fuzz ball on the back of my head the size of a soccer ball and I smelt of sick! My friend Jo, suggested that that was the normal look for any Essex girl after a night on the piss in Romford!!!!!!

I have shattered all hospital records for the time that my treatment took—every time the nurses enter the room and the machine goes off, the time they spend until they leave gets added to my 48 hours so that you get the correct amount of treatment—Dr Doll was not expecting me to be done until at least 6pm Friday night. She high fived me and gave me a hug (even though I looked and smelt appallingly bad) saying I had been a model patient and was very brave. I completed my treatment plan of 47.79 hours in 50 hours and 18 minutes.

I will find out soon if I have the all clear, my appointment is on January 12th, 10.30 for a scan and then 1pm to see Dr Doll and get the results. So let's all keep our fingers crossed and get the champagne ready.

As I type this e-mail, it is Saturday night and I am very achy (not sure if that's a real word!) and a bit sore. I have got cream to apply to my bed sores, my mouth ulcers seem a bit better today and I am looking forward to getting the Christmas decorations up this week.

Happy birthday to Michele for tomorrow, congratulations to my friend who is pregnant (I won't name her as I don't know if she told anyone yet![3]) thank you

---

3.   My friend Anita later gave birth to a beautiful, healthy boy called Rhys.

Clint & Andrea for a lovely dinner last Saturday, happy 40th to my brother in law Jason and Kelly, I hope the fire didn't do too much damage!!!!

Lots of love to you all, I will be in touch next week,

Louise xxxxxxxxx

Martin had decided that in order to make me feel better, he would bring my nicest clothes and jewelry to the hospital so that I could go home feeling like a princess. It was a wonderful gesture and had I not stunk to high heaven and had an enormous matted fur ball on the back of my head, I might just have managed to pull it off. Unfortunately, I looked a bit like a hooker who hadn't washed in a fortnight!

Subject: Just checking in!
Date: Tuesday, December 13, 2005

Hi everyone,

Just wanted to let you all know how I am, it's been 2 weeks today since my final radiation and I am feeling stronger every day. I still get very tired and have to have a sleep most afternoons but physically I feel 100% and I am sure that the cancer has gone for good.

I am not going back to work until Jan 9th so we are enjoying our time without hospital visits. Today we bought a meat grinder and made some sausages!!!! They turned out really well and we had sausage, egg and chips for tea!

Martin was overdue for his cancer check up and had a full medical today. Everything was fine and the doctor was pleased to report him healthy!

My mum arrives here on Saturday for a 2 week stay and as you can imagine, we have a lot to celebrate this Christmas. I don't really know what else to say except Merry Christmas and happy, healthy new year to you all!

I am pursuing the idea of writing a book using the emails that we have exchanged as a base so will let you know how that progresses.

Love Louise xx

Subject: ALL CLEAR!!!!!
Date: Thursday, January 12, 2006

Hi everyone,

I went to the hospital for my appointment today my cancer is not there any more! I felt very strange when Dr Doll was telling me, I expected to be elated or emotional but I really didn't feel much at all. Martin thinks that it was probably because I was so sure that the cancer had gone, I wasn't being told anything that I didn't already know. I did celebrate with a half a bottle of gin so please excuse any typos!

Obviously I am relieved that I am well again and I am pleased that my doctor will keep a close eye on me, I have some inflamed scar tissue on my cervix and have an appointment for a Pap smear in February to check that everything is proceeding normally and will also get appointments for a bone density and CT scan within the next 4 or 5 weeks.

I have been getting a lot of pins and needles in my hands and feet during the night and when I mentioned it today it is caused by the high levels of toxins that the chemo deposits in your body, the only other problems that we discussed today were about my hips getting stiff—which is inflammation caused by radiotherapy, and tiredness again just a normal side effect.

I returned to work on Tuesday but am struggling a bit with full days. Dr Doll said today that she doesn't want me back at work for at least 4 weeks (will chat with you about that tomorrow James!) and was horrified when I said I had already been back to work! Obviously I feel able to work otherwise I wouldn't have gone back so soon but I will have to only do what I can as I don't want to make myself ill.

Not sure if I already mentioned it but Martin passed his reflexology exams so is now a qualified therapist!

Well it's 9.55pm and way past my bedtime so I am off now, thank you all for your very supportive emails, they really did help me get through the tough times.

Love Louise xx

Subject: Hi
Date: Sunday, January 22, 2006

Hi everyone,

Thought you might like to see some pictures that we took last Thursday. We went snow shoeing to Kananaskis in our efforts to keep fit! We managed to complete a 5km trail fairly easily and took some lovely photos of the scenery.

I am working just 3 days a week (Mon, Wed & Fri) for the next month and am hoping that my employers like the arrangement as much as I do and will hopefully change my contract to make it a permanent thing!

Hope you are all keeping well,

Louise x

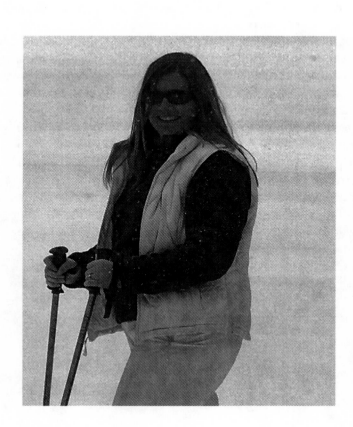

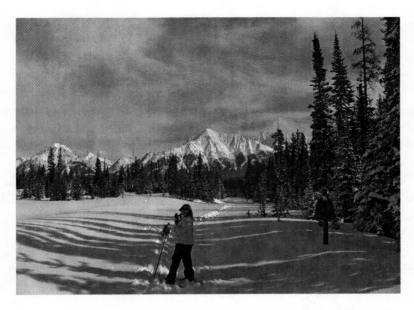

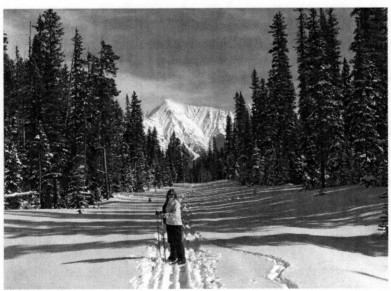

Subject: health update
Date: Sunday, February 12, 2006

Hi everyone,

Before I start, I have added some new people to this list as I have spoken to a couple of friends from the UK this week that seemed to be under the impression that I am a suffering, crying mess!! I know I can't be in contact with every single person I know but I don't want people worrying about me unnecessarily.

I had my check up on Thursday with Dr Doll; she was very pleased with me but couldn't do a smear test yet as the treated area is still quite inflamed. She is booking me in for an MRI scan which should give her very detailed info regarding the scar area; I am also having a CT scan on Feb 28th and go back for my next check up in 6 weeks time.

My bone density scan wasn't very good, it was a base line test as the radiation and menopause won't have affected my bones just yet, apparently my bones are in the low, normal range which would be fine on an average person, but as mine are going to deteriorate over the next year because of my treatment, I have to address this as quite an urgent problem! Dr Doll advised that in these circumstances she would prescribe HRT but as she knows that I am not keen on taking that route, she has made me an appointment at the osteoporosis clinic. They will have a better understanding of what is likely to happen to my bones and will also be able to properly assess my risk for osteoporosis. I felt very disappointed that my bones weren't strong and healthy; I had just assumed that they would be great! As a child, I didn't drink milk or eat yoghurt or cheese; I guess I'm paying for that now.

My blood tests confirmed that I am post menopausal and my symptoms should only last for about 6 months at the absolute most. The only symptoms that I get are 2 or 3 hot flushes a day and they are very manageable. Everyone has been very surprised that I don't seem to be getting mood swings or tearful, irritable days. Maybe it's all the reflexology that is helping!

I am still working 3 days a week and Dr Doll was very insistent that I shouldn't do more than that at this stage, the radiation dose that I was given was quite high and continues to affect you for quite some time after the treatment ends. My employers have been fine about me working part time—time wise, I couldn't have picked a better time to be off sick as my employer lost his job around the time of my diagnosis so has been able to stay home with the children while I concentrate on my recovery—although I only get paid for the days I work and I didn't get paid anything at all when I was off work, at least I don't feel beholden to them.

When we are at the hospital I always go back to my radiation room and chemo suite to say hi to the nurses, it makes me feel very sad when I see obvious first timers in the waiting areas, they look so scared and I just want to tell everyone that it'll be fine, look at me, I was in your position only 5 months ago! I am hoping that if my book idea takes off, it will be available to the hospital for newly diagnosed patients; I wish there had been something like that for me. I have been reading some of the e-mails that I sent to you all in the first few weeks after my diagnosis and I can't believe how scared I was. When you see what can be done in such amazing hospitals like the Tom Baker, you realize that a positive cancer diagnosis is not necessarily a death sentence.

On that note, I am signing off for now. Anyone who is receiving this for the first time and would like to read any of my other updates, let me know, I have copies!

Lots of love Louise xxxxx

Subject: More good news!
Date: Sunday March 12, 2006

Hi everyone,

we have just returned from a fantastic week away, as a thank you for looking after me present for Martin, I booked for us to stay in Kananaskis at a lodge called Mount Engadine. The lodge is at the base of the mountains and as you can see from the pictures, is very beautiful.

We wanted to get away and chill for a while after our cancer nightmare and this was a perfect week. It was sunny every day and there was lots of snow. We snow shoed up a mountain trail and reached a height of 6840feet, we also tried cross country skiing for the first time which was hilarious and a lot harder than it looks! Just about the only thing that didn't ache was my hair!

On the subject of hair, I have lots of new hair growing through so my hair is a real mess as I can't get it to lay flat, I look like I have a hair halo—very odd!!! Not complaining though, I remember how I felt when I thought I might lose it all.

Sunday morning

I forgot that I didn't finish this e-mail!!! So yesterday we hiked 14 km up to a mountain ridge called powder face and beat our previous high by 40 feet—I think that clearly proves that I am feeling very well and am actually fitter now than before my cancer. My legs ache a bit this morning but so do Martin's!

I have decided to get another tattoo (sorry mum) and want to incorporate one of the tattoo's that the radiation department gave me—I am unsure what to get at the moment so would be grateful for any ideas. Kat Von D is an amazing tattoo artist from the States who is visiting the Calgary tattoo festival this September and I have e-mailed her to get an appointment so I have a bit of time to decide what to get!

Well I will sign off now as I am hopefully going to chat with Jamie & Daniel over the webcam in a minute. Keep well everyone,

Love Louise xxx

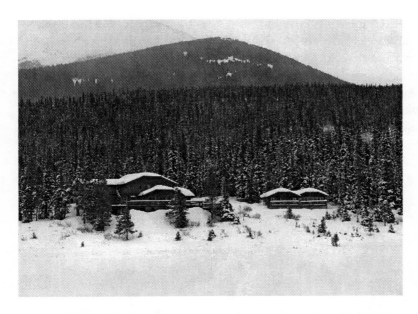

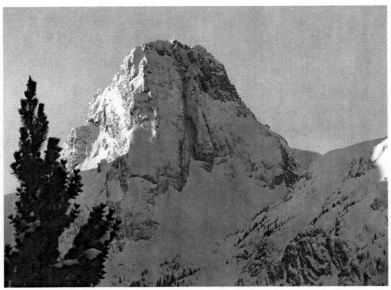

I booked a week away to Engadine Lodge as a surprise for Martin to say thank you for looking after me so well. Even though I hadn't worked for four months so hadn't earned any money, I really needed a break too. It's quite amazing how those daily trips to the hospital for radiation, tire you out. You are literally in the radiation unit for a maximum of fifteen minutes each day but because your appointments are at different times each day, everything you do has to be planned around that time. As time goes on, the radiation itself tires you out and consequently by the end of your treatment, you are truly exhausted.

Subject: good news again!!!!!!
Date: Sunday, March 12, 2006

I forgot to include the good news in the e-mail I just sent! Obviously I was typing using my menopause brain!!!!!!

The good news is my MRI & CT scans both came back clear—Dr Doll is obviously pleased and I was speechless, upset and ecstatic all at the same time. Martin's blood tests for his tumor markers were also fine so we are both cancer free.

Sorry for the confusion, I can't believe I forgot to include the actual subject of the email!

Love Louise x

We arrived back from our week away and while Martin unpacked the car, I went inside to make a drink. I listened to the answer phone messages, the first one being from Dr Doll. She basically said that she was very pleased with my test results and that there was no evidence of cancer anywhere in my body. I burst into tears and ran downstairs to tell Martin, unfortunately the only words that he understood through my sobbing, were Dr Doll and cancer. Once I had calmed down enough to explain properly and Martin had listened to the message himself, we were obviously elated.

We have kept that message on our answer phone and when ever I feel upset or annoyed about anything, I play the message and it instantly brings a smile to my face.

Subject: Update
Date: Thursday, March 30, 2006 (Martin's birthday)

Hi everyone,

I have been to see Dr Doll today for a check up and to have a Pap smear (the first one since my diagnosis). Having the test wasn't particularly pleasant but Dr Doll was really pleased with my progress and could see a definite improvement in the redness and scar tissue. I will know the results in about a week so will let you all know, this is the final test and the one that I am most worried about because it is looking at individual cells that can't be seen on a CT or MRI scan—fingers crossed!!!!

The doctor also assessed my fitness levels and has requested that I continue working only 3 days a week at least until my next appointment in 6 weeks time (sorry James!) I asked her about my hair—which is growing like mad and is very thick and unmanageable—and she confirmed what I already thought, my cells that were killed off by the chemo and radiation are growing back and replacing themselves and because my body is so healthy at the moment, I have lots of extra nutrients to feed my hair and fingernails!

I have decided to try and raise some money for the Tom Baker cancer centre and on April 22nd will attempt to climb the 802 steps to the top of the Calgary tower—the average healthy person could apparently complete this feat in about 20 minutes. I am not sure if I will be able to make it but have applied for the official sponsor forms from the Alberta Cancer Board and once I have them, I will be asking all of you to sponsor me and help me to thank the Tom Baker Cancer centre for saving my life. Dr Doll has said she will sponsor me and has been very encouraging.

My book is also progressing nicely and Dr Doll said she would be honored to write the foreword for me when I asked her today.

On a lighter note, Martin is now calling me Chewbacca (star wars) because of my hair—not at all flattering but sadly true!

I will be in touch soon with sponsor details and hopefully good results from my smear test. I also wanted to say thank you to all of you who went for a smear test at my request. Three of you had positive results but all are ok after further checks. I will be reminding you when you need to go again!!!!!

Bye for now

Louise x

Subject: Cancer free!
Date: Tuesday, April 11, 2006

Hi all,

Great news, my first Pap smear since my treatment was negative!!!!!! I no longer have cancer. We are obviously relieved and on cloud nine at the moment. I am so grateful to my doctors for curing me and to Martin for looking after me so well and to all of you for your support through this testing time.

I have contacted the Alberta Cancer Board and they have agreed to accept Visa or MasterCard donations via their secure website for anyone who wishes to sponsor my Calgary tower walk. I would be so grateful if you could all pledge something, however small—it all goes to a good cause. I am hoping to raise $1000 for the Tom Baker Cancer Centre. Martin is going to climb the steps with me and has said he will get me to the top even if he has to carry me on his back!! Let's hope that he doesn't have to do that or I will be asking for donations to buy him a back brace!!!!!

The link for donations is: http://www.cancerboard.ab.ca/foundation/donations.htm

Please make sure that you fill in

Event name: Calgary tower walk.
Participant name: Louise Lampard

The question that says "please use my gift for...." choose patient programs & special incentives and then choose Tom Baker Cancer Centre. This will ensure that all the money I raise will go directly to the hospital unit that treated me.

The above info is needed so that I can see who has sponsored me and keep a note of how much I have raised. You can either pay now regardless of how I do or you can wait to see if I complete the walk on the 22nd and then donate. The cancer board has asked that all donations be received by them no later than 30 days after the event.

I have attached a picture of the tower I will be climbing for those of you who haven't visited us yet!

Please, please help me to raise $1000 to thank the doctors for saving my life. If any of you lot in the UK have trouble with the online donations, you can always send me a bankers draft or travelers cheques in Canadian dollars, made payable to: The Alberta Cancer Board. I noticed on the donation page that it mentions donating from within Canada only, I have been assured that you can just ignore that but if you have any problems, please let me know.

My book is progressing nicely and Dr Doll (who is sponsoring me on my walk!) has agreed to write the foreword for me—I promise I won't make you buy my book if you agree to sponsor me!!!!!!! Someone has already pointed out that you won't need to buy my book—you already know everything that will be in it!!!!!!

Thank you all so much for supporting me,

Love Louise xxxx

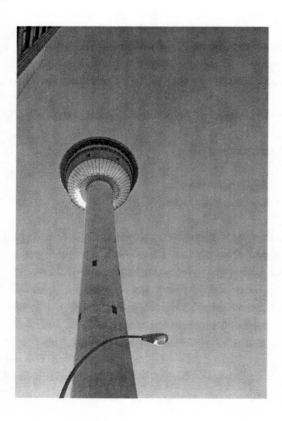

Subject: sponsorship
Date: Wednesday, April 19, 2006

Hi all,

We seem to have had a breakdown in communication!!!! The cancer board is now saying that they can only accept donations from within Canada! I am not sure what the solution is—I will contact them and find out if they will accept sterling cheques and let you all know. Otherwise if one of you would like to volunteer, I can get everyone to send their sponsor money to one person who could transfer the money to a Canadian draft and post it to me????

I will be in touch,

Love Louise xxxx

Subject: Calgary tower walk
Date: Wednesday, April 19, 2006

Hi all,

My sister has volunteered to collect UK sponsorship so I will forward you all her details shortly. If you can send her cheques, she will organise a Canadian bank draft and send it to the cancer board.

I will send an e-mail with Melanie's details in a minute,

Thanks Louise xx

Subject: Calgary tower
Date: Saturday, April 22, 2006

I did it!!

It has been a really crappy day, wet and snowy so we didn't rush to get downtown to the tower very early. We started the climb at 12.15pm and I broke out in a sweat by stair number 35!!! Not a good start! My determination kept me going until stair 405, when I was overtaken by a girl on her 15th trip up the stairs; I had to fight off the instinct to trip her up!

We made it to the top in 22 minutes—not bad even if I do say so myself

Apparently the average healthy person takes 20 minutes so I was really pleased to have completed the climb in 22.

Because today has been so overcast, the views from the top weren't that great so we took the elevator back down and collected our free t-shirt. It was actually a bit of an anti climax, the stair well was small and bland with no views, so I am hoping to raise lots of money in order to have made it worth while!

My sister is going to keep a record of all the money she collects (none so far!) so I will let you all know how much you helped me to raise.

I am off to soak my muscles in the bath now!

Love Louise x

Subject: Health update
Date: Thursday, June 22, 2006

Hi everyone,

Just a short update, I have just returned from my second check up and all appears to be well, Dr Doll has done another Pap smear as well as the usual blood tests and chest x-ray—results will be back late next week! She had a good poke around and assured me that she was very pleased with my progress—my cervix is apparently very loose and before you all take the piss—it's supposed to be loose!!!! It basically means that the scarring caused by radiation is minimal. She has ordered another MRI scan to be done—not sure when, and I have another appointment to see her on Sept 14th.

I can't tell you how pleased I am to report that I raised over $1500 doing my Calgary tower walk. Thank you all so much for sponsoring me, I have attached a picture of me handing over the cheque to Dr Doll today. So many of you in the UK sent money, I am so grateful and will e-mail you all individually to thank you, also I would like to thank my Canadian supporters, Andrea & Clint, Karen & Peter, Barry & Cynthia and Michele & James for sending money directly to the cancer board in my name.

I also wanted to let you all know that we are leaving next Friday morning for a road trip and will be unable to access our e-mails or home phone until August 7th. We will have Martin's cell phone with us for emergencies but are looking forward to a nice long break!

Hope you are all as well as we are, I will be in touch soon

Lots of love Louise xxx

p.s happy 60th George Rudgley

Subject: thank you
Date: Sunday, June 25, 2006

Hi all,

I just wanted to say a big thank you to you all for sponsoring me. I had initially hoped to raise a thousand dollars but with your help, I raised over $2000 for the Tom Baker cancer centre here in Calgary.

Thanks also to Iris's swimming friends, Tony & Jean, Martin's aunt Eileen, Kim's sister Anita and Trudi and Tracie, I don't have current e-mail addresses for them but hopefully you can pass on my thanks.

Also thanks to my sister, Melanie for collecting the money and organising a Canadian bank draft.

Hope you all have a great summer; I will be in touch when we return from our vacation in August.

Love Louise xx

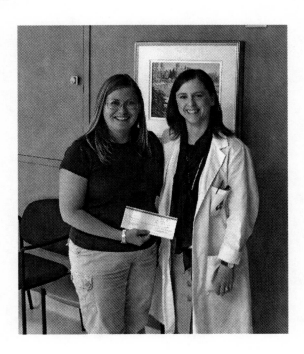

5

One Year Later

Subject: A year already!
Date: Sunday, November 19, 2006

Hi everyone,

I know it's been a long time since I wrote to you all (not including my e-mail encouraging you to buy my calendar on www.lulu.com!) but I wanted to send you all a little reminder. Fast approaching is the one year anniversary of the end of my treatment. I know a lot of you will already have booked your Pap smear check ups but for those who haven't, please call your doctors now. Also for all the males reading this and feeling rather smug—if you are over 40 (and we know most of you are!!!!) then it is time for you to get a prostate exam done.

Please, please remember how simple these examinations are compared to the treatment you might have to have for an undetected cancer.

I have nearly finished my book. I am hoping to take a draft copy to my next appointment with Dr Doll. She has agreed to correct any medical terminology that I might have got wrong and also will be writing the foreword. I will be using everyone's first names only in the book and will obviously not be printing any of your e-mail addresses or contact details. If anyone wants their name changed then please let me know. Equally if any of you have a hankering to be famous, I can just as easily print your full name, phone number, measurements, and a photo!

As for me, I am pretty much back to normal now. I am working full time again and we hit the slopes of Sunshine yesterday for our first ski of the season—I wiped out pretty spectacularly so I have nowhere to go but up! I am off now to nurse my bruises

I look forward to hearing all of your news and hope that everyone has clear test results! One last thing, last year as a direct result of my cancer diagnosis, 41 of my female friends went for a Pap smear test, four of you had problems needing further investigation. Thankfully the end result was good for all of you. Please keep that in mind and tell as many people that you can about the importance of yearly Pap smears. (For everyone in the UK—three yearly testing is not enough, pay and go privately if you have to).

Love to you all,

Louise xxx

6

Early Menopause

I believed rather naively that entering my menopause aged 35 would really be the least of my worries. Friends had shared with me the delight of no more periods or birth control and I have to admit I agreed with them, that was until I suffered my first hot flush!

The hot flushes were the only tangible symptom of menopause for me and in the beginning they were relentless. I would find myself stripping off clothing during mealtimes (I took a few people by surprise! Just kidding) and during the night, I was either too hot or too cold. It felt as though I had lost the ability to regulate my body temperature.

As you all know by now, I am not the sort of person to take drugs unnecessarily and I had decided, against medical advice, to learn all that I could about early menopause and pick up any self help tips to see if I could survive the menopause naturally. Dr Doll was more than willing to help me and I assured her that if, after my bone scan, it was important for me to take HRT for healthy bones, then I would go ahead and take medication.

My bone scan wasn't actually that great but the osteoporosis clinic agreed that with plenty of exercise and the right diet, I should be able to proceed with my 'natural' approach.

Almost immediately it became apparent that foods high in either sugar or more particularly salt would bring on a hot flush instantly.

We avoided both as much as we could and made sure that I ate plenty of salmon, tuna and fresh fruits and vegetables every day. Vitamin D is vital as is enables the body to absorb calcium more efficiently. We both always enjoyed cooking and now make sure that we make everything from scratch, mainly to ensure that we avoid the foods and ingredients that cause me to suffer hot flushes.

Soon fizzy drinks joined the 'no' list as did caffeine, pizza and anything processed. Luckily alcohol and chocolate don't seem to have a negative effect!

Very soon I was back in control and with my master chef Martin at the helm; we were controlling my symptoms nicely. As a special favor to Dr Doll, I fell off the 'food wagon' once or twice and indulged in junk food in order to prove that the menopause diet really was working! Within a few minutes of eating salt, in particular, I get very severe hot flushes and feel ill almost to the point of fainting. We have become vigilant at checking labels and ingredients to ensure that we are not putting unnecessary chemicals into our bodies. If the food we wish to purchase has an unpronounceable ingredient, it definitely goes back on the shelf as does anything with more than 1 or 2 grams of salt per 100 grams. Along with salt, anything that has added colors or any E numbers has an almost immediately, adverse effect.

I have to visit the bone density clinic again in two years time for a comparison scan and I am obviously hoping that having done everything that was asked of me, my bones will not have deteriorated and I will not have to take hormone replacements.

I have shared my diet findings with a number of friends who have been suffering menopause symptoms, and all have agreed that they feel so much better and importantly, feel that they have more control over their health and well being.

7

A Husband's Point of View

Standing in Dr M's office I was suddenly aware of the word "cancer" and although Louise and I had considered the possibility I had convinced myself that she had fibroids and that confirmation of this condition would immediately alleviate us of the worry and fears of the last couple of weeks allowing us to continue with our lives.

I felt as though I had been hit by a truck, my whole mind and body reeled with the shock of what I had just heard, I felt nausea, faint, detached from everything and everybody in the room except Louise.

I wanted this to be a mistake; I didn't want Louise to be ill.

I just wanted to take Louise into my arms, cuddle her and assure her that everything would be ok.

I felt utterly helpless, what could I say? What could I do? I knew that we wouldn't wake in the morning only to find this had been a horrendous nightmare (little did I know then but sleep would elude us for many weeks only compounding the horror of our situation)

We left the hospital in a state of shock, fear and disbelief, I had never felt so low in my life, my brain had only one focus and that was the word "cancer" and all it entailed.

I don't remember driving home or whether we were offered a prognosis at the hospital, I felt as though my head would explode with worry.

At some point during the initial post diagnosis period I suddenly realized that however terrible and pitiful I was feeling, Louise would be feeling a hundred times worse, a hundred times more frightened, a hundred times more alone with her illness, and that even if I could do nothing to physically aid her recovery; I could at least do everything within my power to make her life easier, reassure her of her doubts, gather information relating to her condition, be strong for her and help her achieve a positive mental attitude.

Rightly or wrongly I felt that this along with the specialist treatment that Louise would receive would be fundamental to aid her recovery.

From a selfish point of view it felt that I had appointed myself a member of her cancer team and with this focused outlook I was in some small way helping with the recovery process which of course helped me. The feeling of uselessness had diminished slightly and had suddenly been replaced with the knowledge that I wasn't just a spectator to this horrible situation, but was indeed in a position to help.

I suddenly considered that one of the reasons that people of my generation are terrified of the word cancer is that it is synonymous with the word death and we therefore have an inherent fear of a disease that we have little understanding.

I then concluded with a strange kind of logic that this could be because of two reasons,

1. As children we were only informed that a family member or person known to us had cancer when they were on their death beds and the subject could no longer be ignored or that,

2. The success rate for a cancer patient was lower when I was a child as the treatment and understanding of the disease was less than it is now.

As far as I was concerned neither of these scenarios applied to Louise and unless I was offered information to the contrary this is what I chose to believe.

This may have seemed a very naive notion but in order to help Louise I would have to glue together some of the fragments of our lives and build a foundation from which to work, and in my own mind by believing my observations this was what I was doing.

I then considered that a lot of the fears that we have as human beings is through ignorance and that the more information relating to both the prognosis and the treatment of the condition we could ascertain the better.

If I could gently persuade Louise of this way of thinking we could work together towards that "positive mental attitude" we so often hear about.

Suddenly from feeling that our lives had been shattered into a million tiny pieces there seemed like there was hope.

Strange as it may seem, from a detached point of view I actually looked forward to Louise's first appointment. I felt that as a team we were doing something positive and that the recovery process had begun, although from a husband's point of view I felt terribly guilty as I knew that I was looking forward to something that would be terrifying for my wife.

It was evident from the very first appointment that we had a fantastic team of people in our corner and that they would be aiming towards a curative treatment and nothing less, but that the months ahead would be stressful, and at times particularly unpleasant.

Of course I had all of the sympathy in the world for Louise and would have willingly traded places with her, as it broke my heart to think of all that she would have to go through but I was starting to see the bigger picture and the life that we would be able to enjoy after the conclusion of the treatment.

Maybe I was selective about what I heard during the hospital visits but I always tried to memorize the positive parts of any consultation as initially I could use this to counteract the fact that Louise had sometimes only absorbed the negative.

I was therefore delighted that within only a couple of visits Louise seemed to be following my lead. I was so proud of her.

Together and with the help of some of the kindest compassionate doctors that we had ever met we had gone from a state of absolute terror, sleepless nights and feeling as though we had no future, to total belief in a curative process and the continuation of our wonderful lives together.

With each visit our confidence grew and because the treatment involved a six week daily hospital visit for treatment it wasn't long before some of the fear of attending had disappeared. It was also reassuring to be interacting with some of the fellow patients that were further down the line with their treatment as they were able to advise us of certain feeling and fears that we may have had but did not want to worry the medical staff with.

It was also reassuring to realize that there are many people living their lives with this illness and with all intents and purpose conducting a perfectly normal life other than the hospital visits.

It is safe to say that nobody would choose to have an illness and have to endure the treatment, worry and heartache synonymous with such a condition.

It has however left both Louise and I with some very memorable and even positive impressions.

Once faced with a life threatening condition and overcoming it you seem to have a completely different life perspective.

The trials and tribulations of everyday life don't seem to hold the same fears and doubts that you once imagined, silly things that once may have seen you get angry rarely matter anymore and life certainly feels more precious to us, with the feeling that it should never be wasted.

We would like to think that having endured what we and millions of other people have, has had a positive effect on us and made us more thoughtful, compassionate people.

In addition, you learn who your true friends are and who you can rely on in times of need, and maybe equally importantly, who you can't.

This comes as somewhat of a revelation as sadly some of those who talked the talk did only that, whereas others, (in some cases people that we barely knew) were fantastic with their support and encouragement, and to those people (I'm sure that you know who you are) I would like to say thank you.

Well I'm delighted to say that we have recently celebrated the one year anniversary of Louise being clear of her illness.

I am immensely grateful to all team members that were instrumental to the success of Louise's treatment.

There are of course no words adequate to show my appreciation for giving me back my beautiful wife.

How can a simple "thank you" be enough?

I think that we sometimes forget that the doctors, nurses, specialists and team members that through their knowledge compassion and dedication allow fellow human beings to continue life touch so many associated lives, for it is not only the patient that continues living but all those that are close to that person.

It is therefore that I not only thank all involved for what they have done for Louise but also for allowing my life to continue with the woman I love.

8

My Cancer Legacy

My life has changed immeasurably over the past year. I have focused a lot of energy on my photography hobby and feel very proud to have published a calendar of my photographs. I have a renewed lust for life and if it were possible to go back in time, I wouldn't change a thing.

My cancer has made me a stronger person and a more compassionate human being.

I feel extremely fortunate to have met some incredible people, cancer patients who smile and fight on regardless and doctors and nurses who give their time selflessly for the good of others.

I could never have survived this experience without the love and support of my wonderful husband, Martin. Having battled his own cancer, we are totally in tune with each other and are so close that it seems at times that we are one person.

Although I was offered counseling to help me come to terms with my cancer, I declined the offer. Unfortunately for my friends and family, I seemed unable to talk about anything except my illness for a whole year! I believe that this must have worked as a therapy for me and I often found myself steering the conversation back to me and my cancer. I am sure I was a huge bore to a lot of people, thoroughly self obsessed and for that I would like to take this opportunity to apologize.

I finally feel that in the last couple of months I have been able to move on and cancer is not the first thing I thing I think about when I wake up in the morning. Although one very sad after effect is the nagging worry that even the most trivial of illnesses, like a cold, will turn out to be far more serious.

I cried more after my treatment ended than I did during my illness. The first time I hiked to the top of Prairie Mountain, Kananaskis, I sobbed like a baby! It felt like such a huge accomplishment.

I feel very proud to have been able to raise over $2000 for the Tom Baker Cancer Centre, Calgary and would like to continue to raise money for them each year.

My confidence really dropped during my treatment and I found it very difficult to make the simplest of decisions. Answering the phone was a nightmare for me; most people didn't know what to say so were very sympathetic in their approach which made me cry instantly. It was easier to deal with more practical people who discussed my situation in a more business like manner. Thankfully my confidence is renewed and I now know that I can do anything I put my mind to. I have faced my mortality and won. I feel invincible and at the same time very aware that death is never far away and I am therefore compelled to get on with enjoying my life to the fullest.

My eyesight worsened as a result of my chemotherapy, apparently that is quite normal—a great excuse to treat myself to a new pair of glasses! My sense of taste has also changed considerably; I no longer crave chocolate, I eat olives all the time (I hated them before) and can now tolerate very spicy food which I never could do before. I have got some on going, minor problems with my hearing, but nothing that I can't deal with.

Mostly, I am not scared of cancer anymore.

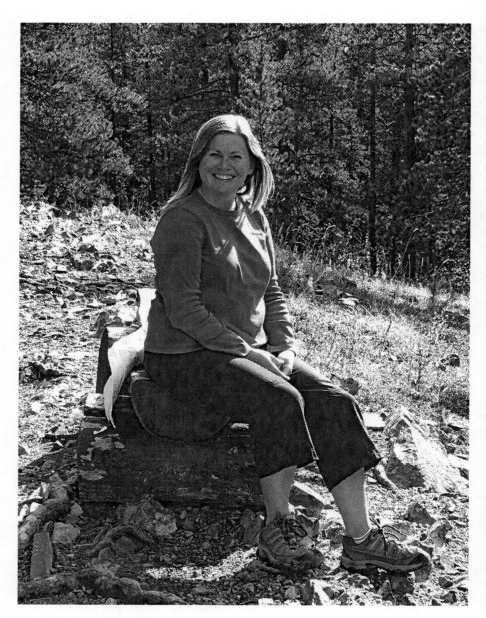

Climbing Prairie Mountain, shortly after finishing cancer treatment.

Epilogue

As this book goes to print, I am almost two years clear of cancer; Martin is five and a half years cancer free.

We are actively raising both money and awareness for the Alberta Cancer Foundation and I am thankful every day to the doctors and nurses who saved my life.

Writing this book has been a wonderful, sad, funny and most of all cathartic experience, I truly believe that a positive mind is the key to survival.

Latest statistics in Alberta show that one in every three Albertans[1] will be diagnosed with cancer in their lifetime; research is the key to a cure. If you would like to donate money to the Alberta Cancer Foundation, you can do so online at www.cancerboard.ab.ca

---

1.   Alberta cancer boards spring 2003 newsletter

Glossary

Biopsy :examination of tissue to be tested for disease

Brachytherapy :a form of radiation therapy

Chemotherapy :the treatment of cancer by chemical substances

Colposcopy :examination of the vagina and neck of the womb

Dysplasia :abnormal growth of tissues

Fibroids :benign fibrous tumor found in the womb

Pap smear :swab of cervical cells to check for abnormalities

Radiotherapy :the treatment of disease by radiation

Radical hysterectomy :surgical removal of womb, ovaries and cervix

Related Websites

www.cancerboard.ab.ca
The Alberta cancer foundation's website, a good start for general cancer info.

www.earlymenopause.com
This website has lots of useful advice for dealing with early menopause.

www.aicr.org.uk
The association for international cancer research.

www.oneless.com
Information about the HPV virus and vaccine.

www.cancer.org
General cancer information from a reliable source.

www.cancerboard.ab.ca/tapestry/
A retreat offered to cancer patients & their families. Run by the ACF.

www.calgarytower.com
This is where I chose to climb and raise money for the ACF

www.mountengadine.com
A beautiful lodge, we stayed there to recuperate after my illness.

www.runningforlife.ca
Website started by my friend Constance to raise money and awareness for cancer.

www.lulu.com
This website publishes and sells a calendar of my photographs.

www.iuniverse.com
My book publishers website.

www.louiselampard.com
My personal site, where you can purchase my photographs and cards.

978-0-595-46081-6
0-595-46081-X

Printed in the United States
127436LV00001B/69/A

9 780595 460816